HIV in the Emergency Department

Guest Editors

MERCEDES TORRES, MD
RACHEL L. CHIN, MD

EMERGENCY MEDICINE CLINICS OF NORTH AMERICA

www.emed.theclinics.com

Consulting Editor
AMAL MATTU, MD

May 2010 • Volume 28 • Number 2

SAUNDERS an imprint of ELSEVIER, Inc.

W.B. SAUNDERS COMPANY

A Division of Elsevier Inc.

1600 John F. Kennedy Boulevard ● Suite 1800 ● Philadelphia, Pennsylvania 19103-2899

http://www.theclinics.com

EMERGENCY MEDICINE CLINICS OF NORTH AMERICA Volume 28, Number 2
May 2010 ISSN 0733-8627, ISBN-13: 978-1-4377-1815-7

Editor: Patrick Manley
Developmental Editor: Theresa Collier

Emergency Medicine Clinics of North America (ISSN 0733-8627) is published quarterly by Elsevier Inc., 360 Park Avenue South, New York, NY, 10010-1710. Months of issue are February, May, August, and November. Business and Editorial Offices: 1600 John F. Kennedy Boulevard, Suite 1800, Philadelphia, PA 19103-2899. Customer Service Office: 6277 Sea Harbor Drive, Orlando, FL 32887-4800. Periodicals postage paid at New York, NY, and additional mailing offices. Subscription prices are $127.00 per year (US students), $247.00 per year (US individuals), $414.00 per year (US institutions), $180.00 per year (international students), $354.00 per year (international individuals), $499.00 per year (international institutions), $180.00 per year (Canadian students), $305.00 per year (Canadian individuals), and $499.00 per year (Canadian institutions). International air speed delivery is included in all *Clinics'* subscription prices. All prices are subject to change without notice. **POSTMASTER:** Send address changes to *Emergency Medicine Clinics of North America*, Elsevier Periodicals Customer Service, 11830 Westline Industrial Drive, St. Louis, MO 63146. Customer Service (orders, claims, online, change of address): Elsevier Periodicals Customer Service, 11830 Westline Industrial Drive, St. Louis, MO 63146. Tel: 1-800-654-2452 (U.S. and Canada); 314-453-7041 (outside U.S. and Canada). Fax: 314-453-5170. E-mail: journalscustomerservice-usa@elsevier.com (for print support); journalsonline support-usa@elsevier.com (for online support).

Reprints. For copies of 100 or more of articles in this publication, please contact the Commercial Reprints Department, Elsevier Inc., 360 Park Avenue South, New York, NY 10010-1710. Tel.: 212-633-3812; Fax: 212-462-1935; E-mail: reprints@elsevier.com.

Emergency Medicine Clinics of North America is covered in *MEDLINE/PubMed (Index Medicus), Current Contents/Clinical Medicine, EMBASE/Excerpta Medica, BIOSIS, SciSearch, CINAHL, ISI/BIOMED,* and *Research Alert.*

Printed and bound by CPI Group (UK) Ltd, Croydon, CR0 4YY
Transferred to Digital Print 2011

Contributors

CONSULTING EDITOR

AMAL MATTU, MD, FAAEM, FACEP
Program Director, Emergency Medicine Residency; Associate Professor, Department of Emergency Medicine, University of Maryland School of Medicine, Baltimore, Maryland

GUEST EDITORS

MERCEDES TORRES, MD
Clinical Assistant Professor, Department of Emergency Medicine, University of Maryland School of Medicine, Baltimore, Maryland

RACHEL L. CHIN, MD
Professor of Emergency Medicine, School of Medicine, University of California, San Francisco; Department of Emergency Medicine, San Francisco General Hospital, San Francisco, California

AUTHORS

GEORGE W. BEATTY, MD, MPH
Associate Clinical Professor of Medicine, University of California, San Francisco, Positive Health Program at San Francisco General Hospital, University of California, San Francisco, San Francisco, California

RACHEL L. CHIN, MD
Professor of Emergency Medicine, School of Medicine, University of California, San Francisco; Department of Emergency Medicine, San Francisco General Hospital, San Francisco, California

CHARLES K. EVERETT, MD
Fellow, Division of Pulmonary and Critical Care Medicine, San Francisco General Hospital, University of California, San Francisco, San Francisco, California

BRENNA M. FARMER, MD
Assistant Professor of Medicine, Attending Physician, Division of Emergency Medicine, Weill-Cornell Medical College, New York Presbyterian Hospital, New York, New York

MATTHEW W. FEI, MD
Attending Pulmonary Physician, Division of Pulmonary and Critical Care Medicine, Bellevue Medical Center, Bellevue, Washington

GREGORY W. HENDEY, MD, FACEP
Vice Chair and Research Director; Professor of Clinical Emergency Medicine, University of California, San Francisco-Fresno Emergency Medicine Residency Program, University of California, San Francisco, Fresno, California

EMILY L. HO, MD, PhD
Clinical Instructor and Fellow, Department of Neurology, University of California, San Francisco; Neurology Service, San Francisco General Hospital, San Francisco, California

SAM S. HSU, MD
Assistant Professor, Department of Emergency Medicine, University of Maryland School of Medicine, Baltimore, Maryland

LAURENCE HUANG, MD
Professor of Clinical Medicine, Divisions of HIV/AIDS and Pulmonary and Critical Care Medicine, San Francisco General Hospital, University of California, San Francisco, San Francisco, California

CHERYL A. JAY, MD
Clinical Professor, Department of Neurology, University of California; Neurology Service, San Francisco General Hospital; Positive Health Program, San Francisco General Hospital, San Francisco, California

MARIAM M. KHAMBATY, MD
Assistant Professor of Medicine, Division of Infectious Disease, University of Maryland School of Medicine, Baltimore, Maryland

STEPHEN Y. LIANG, MD
Clinical Fellow, Division of Infectious Diseases, Barnes-Jewish Hospital, Washington University School of Medicine, Saint Louis, Missouri

DANIEL M. LUGASSY, MD
Medical Toxicology Fellow, New York City Poison Control Center, New York University School of Medicine, New York, New York

RAKESH K. MISHRA, MD, FACC
Berkeley Cardiovascular Medical Group, Berkeley, California

SIAMAK MOAYEDI, MD
Assistant Professor, Department of Emergency Medicine, School of Medicine, University of Maryland, Elkridge, Maryland

LEWIS S. NELSON, MD
Director, Fellowship in Medical Toxicology; Associate Professor, Department of Emergency Medicine, New York City Poison Control Center, New York University School of Medicine, New York, New York

E. TURNER OVERTON, MD
Assistant Professor of Medicine, Division of Infectious Diseases, Barnes-Jewish Hospital, Washington University School of Medicine, Saint Louis, Missouri

SARA B. SCOTT, MD
Instructor, Department of Emergency Medicine, University of Maryland School of Medicine, Baltimore, Maryland

WESLEY H. SELF, MD
Assistant Professor, Department of Emergency Medicine, Vanderbilt University; Veterans Affairs National Quality Scholars Fellow, Tennessee Valley Healthcare System, Veterans Health Administration, Nashville, Tennessee

SUKHJIT S. TAKHAR, MD
Assistant Clinical Professor of Emergency Medicine, University of California, San Francisco-Fresno Emergency Medicine Residency Program, University of California, San Francisco; Faculty, Division of Infectious Disease, University of California, San Francisco, Fresno, California

MERCEDES TORRES, MD
Clinical Assistant Professor, Department of Emergency Medicine, University of Maryland School of Medicine, Baltimore, Maryland

Contents

Emergency medicine physicians are uniquely positioned to detect manifestations of human immunodeficiency virus (HIV) disease in the head and neck region. Awareness of the myriad of opportunistic infections and malignancies that involve the head, neck, and eyes is paramount to their diagnosis and treatment. On occasion some of these manifestations are a direct result of HIV and represent the initial signs of primary HIV infection. In some cases, prompt diagnosis and therapy will lead to preservation of function and prevention of significant morbidity.

The aspects of cardiovascular disease in the patient infected with HIV that are of particular relevance to the emergency physician, including coronary artery disease and acute coronary syndromes, pericardial disease, and dilated cardiomyopathy are discussed in this review.

Respiratory complaints are a common reason for patients with HIV infection to present to an emergency department (ED). "HIV and shortness of breath" is one of the most frequent chief complaints on ED triage sheets, and the differential diagnosis is broad. Pulmonary etiologies include infectious and noninfectious causes that are related and unrelated to underlying HIV infection and range from the minor to the life threatening. This article focuses on respiratory emergencies among HIV-infected patients and discusses their typical presentation and diagnostic evaluation as well as therapeutic interventions that should be initiated in an ED.

Diarrhea is an exceedingly common complaint in patients with human immunodeficiency virus (HIV) infection, and the severity of symptoms ranges from mild, self-limiting diarrhea to debilitating disease that can result in malnutrition, volume loss, and shock. Up to 40% of patients with HIV infection report at least 1 episode of diarrhea in a given month, and approximately 1 quarter of patients experience chronic diarrhea at some point. The prevalence of diarrhea increases with decreasing CD4 counts. The clinical features, diagnosis, and management of diarrhea in patients with HIV are reviewed.

HIV-infected patients are vulnerable to developing altered mental status (AMS) for myriad reasons, including the effects of HIV itself, the accompanying immune dysfunction, associated systemic illness, comorbid psychiatric disorders, and complicated medication regimens. Combination antiretroviral therapy (ART) has decreased the incidence of central nervous system (CNS) opportunistic infections (OIs) and HIV-associated dementia, but the benefits are not absolute. In addition to CNS OIs and complications of complex multisystem disease, immune reconstitution events developing in the early weeks and months after initiating ART may affect the brain and cause AMS. This article examines the epidemiology, diagnosis, and currently available treatment for patients with HIV-related AMS.

This article discusses the various hematologic and oncologic diseases to consider when caring for a patient with HIV infection. These diseases are not only more common in this patient population, but they can often be more severe, leading to greater morbidity and mortality than would be expected for a patient without HIV infection. Among the hematologic conditions discussed are common blood dyscrasias such as anemia, leucopenia, and thrombocytopenia, as well as less common disease processes such as immune thrombocytopenic purpura, thrombotic thrombocytopenic purpura, and venous thromboses. The oncologic diseases discussed include AIDS-defining conditions, such as Kaposi sarcoma, invasive cervical carcinoma and non-Hodgkin lymphoma. The recognition of these conditions in patients infected with HIV is of paramount importance for identifying patients at high risk of morbidity and mortality.

There are several musculoskeletal conditions that are specific or unique to the patient infected with human immunodeficiency virus (HIV). These conditions affecting the patient with HIV can be divided into 4 categories: disseminated diseases, bone disorders, joint disease, and myopathies. This review focuses on the manifestations of HIV on musculoskeletal disease as they relate to the emergency physician.

Antiretroviral therapy has revolutionized the care of individuals infected with the human immunodeficiency virus (HIV) and has fundamentally altered the scope of the disease. Acute renal failure and chronic kidney disease from medication toxicity and comorbid noninfectious illnesses are just as likely today as end-organ injury from the virus itself. Chronic immunosuppression renders HIV-infected patients vulnerable to any of several unique urological infections not frequently seen in immunocompetent patients. A deeper understanding of renal and urological emergencies in the context of the HIV-infected patient will better prepare the emergency physician to render optimal care to this rapidly expanding and aging patient population.

Cutaneous diseases occur in most people infected with human immunodeficiency virus (HIV) and at a higher rate than people not infected with HIV. Common HIV-related rashes and rashes made unusual by HIV infection are reviewed.

In 2001 and then again in 2006, the Centers for Disease Control and Prevention (CDC) published guidelines recommending universal HIV screening in acute care settings, including emergency departments (EDs). The value of early identification and treatment of HIV-infected patients is clear, but the most effective method for accomplishing this has yet to be determined. In this article, published experiences by ED-based HIV screening programs are reviewed to learn lessons from their mistakes and accomplishments. The goal of this article is to encourage thought regarding previous experiences with HIV screening and future ideas for improving efforts to this end. By examining the variety of HIV testing kits available, the debate regarding targeted testing versus screening, the consent and patient education requirements, and the staffing models used to implement HIV testing in the ED, this review aims to provide emergency physicians and administrators with options that can be tailored based on the resources available in their specific venue.

Acute human immunodeficiency virus (HIV) infection, also known as primary HIV infection, is the initial phase of infection, spanning from inoculation to the establishment of CD4 count and viral load set points. This phase is marked by dynamic changes in viral replication and host immune responses and contains 2 important clinical events: acute retroviral syndrome and seroconversion. Acute HIV infection is challenging to diagnose, but with recent improvements in diagnostic testing and a heightened awareness of acute HIV, the emergency physician is well positioned to make this diagnosis and initiate important interventions for the individual patient and public health.

Immune reconstitution inflammatory syndrome (IRIS) must be considered in the differential diagnosis for any patient infected with HIV who has begun ART in the preceding months. Distinguishing between manifestations of IRIS and active infection is of paramount importance and poses a diagnostic challenge to the provider in the acute care setting. Presentations of IRIS are often atypical for the precipitating pathogen, and novel presentations are likely. Of the diseases associated with IRIS, mycobacteria and cryptococcal infections are commonly encountered, as are dermatologic symptoms in general. The most clinically significant complications of IRIS are those involving the central nervous system, lungs, and eye, and in many of these scenarios systemic steroids may be of benefit. Management should rarely include interruption of ART, except possibly in severe, life-threatening complications.

Although antiretroviral therapy (ART) for human immunodeficiency virus (HIV) has been in use since 1987, the initiation of highly active ART has produced an increase in adverse drug reactions. This is a new challenge as many of the adverse drug reactions attributable to ART may be indistinguishable from non–drug-related illnesses. The emergency physician must be aware of the potential complications of ART as affected patients may present with nonspecific symptoms. The focus of this article is the metabolic and hepatobiliary adverse effects of ART.

Health care workers are at risk for human immunodeficiency virus (HIV) and other infectious pathogens through exposure to blood and body fluids. Antiretroviral medications have been prescribed for postexposure prophylaxis following occupational exposure to the HIV since the early 1990s. This practice has since been extended to nonoccupational situations, such as sexual assaults. The efficacy of prophylactic therapy may be highly time-dependent and should be initiated as soon as possible. Wound care management and referral for social, medical, or advocacy services remain important for all cases.

RELATED INTEREST

Heart Failure Clinics, January 2009, Vol. 5, No. 1 (pages 1–148)
Management of Heart Failure in the Emergent Situation
James F. Neuenschwander, MD, FACEP and W. Frank Peacock, MD, FACEP,
Guest Editors

THE CLINICS ARE NOW AVAILABLE ONLINE!

Access your subscription at:
www.theclinics.com

GOAL STATEMENT

The goal of *Emergency Medicine Clinics of North America* is to keep practicing physicians up to date with current clinical practice in emergency medicine by providing timely articles reviewing the state of the art in patient care.

ACCREDITATION

The *Emergency Medical Clinics of North America* is planned and implemented in accordance with the Essential Areas and Policies of the Accreditation Council for Continuing Medical Education (ACCME) through the joint sponsorship of the University of Virginia School of Medicine and Elsevier. The University of Virginia School of Medicine is accredited by the ACCME to provide continuing medical education for physicians.

The University of Virginia School of Medicine designates this educational activity for a maximum of 15 *AMA PRA Category 1 Credits™* for each issue, 60 credits per year. Physicians should only claim credit commensurate with the extent of their participation in the activity.

The American Medical Association has determined that physicians not licensed in the US who participate in this CME activity are eligible for a maximum of 15 *AMA PRA Category 1 Credits™* for each issue, 60 credits per year.

The Emergency Medicine Clinics of North America CME program is approved by the American College of Emergency Physicians for 60 hours of ACEP Category I Credit per year.

Credit can be earned by reading the text material, taking the CME examination online at http://www.theclinics.com/home/cme, and completing the evaluation. After taking the test, you will be required to review any and all incorrect answers. Following completion of the test and evaluation, your credit will be awarded and you may print your certificate.

FACULTY DISCLOSURE/CONFLICT OF INTEREST

The University of Virginia School of Medicine, as an ACCME accredited provider, endorses and strives to comply with the Accreditation Council for Continuing Medical Education (ACCME) Standards of Commercial Support, Commonwealth of Virginia statutes, University of Virginia policies and procedures, and associated federal and private regulations and guidelines on the need for disclosure and monitoring of proprietary and financial interests that may affect the scientific integrity and balance of content delivered in continuing medical education activities under our auspices.

The University of Virginia School of Medicine requires that all CME activities accredited through this institution be developed independently and be scientifically rigorous, balanced and objective in the presentation/discussion of its content, theories and practices.

All authors/editors participating in an accredited CME activity are expected to disclose to the readers relevant financial relationships with commercial entities occurring within the past 12 months (such as grants or research support, employee, consultant, stock holder, member of speakers bureau, etc.). The University of Virginia School of Medicine will employ appropriate mechanisms to resolve potential conflicts of interest to maintain the standards of fair and balanced education to the reader. Questions about specific strategies can be directed to the Office of Continuing Medical Education, University of Virginia School of Medicine, Charlottesville, Virginia.

The faculty and staff of the University of Virginia Office of Continuing Medical Education have no financial affiliations to disclose.

The authors/editors listed below have identified no professional or financial affiliations for themselves or their spouse/partner:
George W. Beatty, MD, MPH; Rachel L. Chin, MD (Guest Editor); Charles K. Everett, MD; Brenna M. Farmer, MD; Matthew W. Fei, MD; Gregory W. Hendey, MD; Emily L. Ho, MD, PhD; Sam S. Hsu, MD; Laurence Huang, MD; Mariam M. Khambaty, MD; Stephen Y. Liang, MD; Daniel M. Lugassy, MD; Patrick Manley (Acquisitions Editor); Amal Mattu, MD, FAAEM, FACEP (Consulting Editor); Siamak Moayedi, MD; Lewis S. Nelson, MD; Sara B. Scott, MD; Wesley H. Self, MD; Sukhjit S. Takhar, MD; Mercedes Torres, MD (Guest Editor); and Bill Woods, MD (Test Author).

The authors/editors listed below have identified the following professional or financial affiliations for themselves of their spouse/partner:
Cheryl A. Jay, MD is employed as a faculty member at UCSF.
Rakesh K. Mishra, MD is on the Speakers' Bureau for ViiV Healthcare.
E. Turner Overton, MD is an industry funded research/investigator, is a consultant, and serves on the Speakers' Bureau for Gilead, Tibotec, and Glaxo-Smith-Kline; serves on the Speakers' Bureau for BMS and Monogram Sciences; and is a consultant and serves on the Speakers' Bureau for Merck and Boehringer Ingelheim.

Disclosure of Discussion of Non-FDA Approved Uses for Pharmaceutical Products and/or Medical Devices.

The University of Virginia School of Medicine, as an ACCME provider, requires that all faculty presenters identify and disclose any off-label uses for pharmaceutical and medical device products. The University of Virginia School of Medicine recommends that each physician fully review all the available data on new products or procedures prior to clinical use.

TO ENROLL

To enroll in the Emergency Medicine Clinics of North America Continuing Medical Education program, call customer service at 1-800-654-2452 or visit us online at www.theclinics.com/home/cme. The CME program is available to subscribers for an additional fee of $195.00.

Foreword

Patients With HIV in the Emergency Department

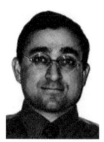

Amal Mattu, MD
Consulting Editor

Since the beginning of mankind, those involved in health care have waged a constant battle against infectious diseases. Early "healers" as well as modern day physicians have struggled to find new therapies to combat deadly microorganisms. Despite many successes, certain infections seem to have thrived, producing pandemics and tremendous international morbidity and mortality. Human immunodeficiency virus, well known simply as HIV, is one such example.

When HIV was first being identified in the 1980s, nobody could have known that this virus would have such a profound influence on so many cultures and societies. The virus has truly proven to have no limits on its victims: men and women as well as adults and children; every nationality has been involved in the virus' rampage. Although a cure has not yet been identified, research has fortunately been able to identify treatments that have controlled the morbidity and mortality rates. Although HIV was once considered a rapid death sentence, it has now become a more chronic disease for many patients through the use of various medication regimens. Because HIV-infected patients are now living longer, the number of these patients presenting to emergency departments is increasing dramatically. More than ever before, it is incumbent on emergency health care providers to be well-versed in managing patients presenting with complications related to HIV as well as in managing patients presenting with a non-HIV–related problem but in whom HIV is a comorbidity.

In this issue of *Emergency Medicine Clinics of North America*, Guest Editors Drs Torres and Chin have assembled an outstanding group of authors to address the challenges we face in caring for patients with HIV in the emergency department. They address HIV-related complications that affect all of the major organ systems, from the skin to the brain. In addition, they address postexposure prophylaxis as well as

Emerg Med Clin N Am 28 (2010) xiii–xiv
doi:10.1016/j.emc.2010.02.002
0733-8627/10/$ – see front matter © 2010 Elsevier Inc. All rights reserved.

emed.theclinics.com

the very important public health topic of rapid HIV screening in the emergency department. Topics also address the more recently described immune reconstitution inflammatory syndrome and the ever-changing issues pertaining to medication side effects. This issue of *Clinics* is a must read for anyone who cares for a significant number of patients with HIV in their emergency department. It represents the most cutting-edge level of knowledge on the topic. Our thanks to Drs Torres, Chin, and their group of authors who have provided this critical information for us all.

Amal Mattu, MD
Department of Emergency Medicine
University of Maryland School of Medicine
110 S. Paca Street, 6th Floor, Suite 200
Baltimore, MD 21201, USA

E-mail address:
amattu@smail.umaryland.edu

Preface

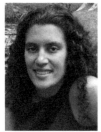 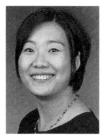

Mercedes Torres, MD   Rachel L. Chin, MD
Guest Editors

Worldwide, an estimated 33 million people are living with human immunodeficiency virus (HIV) infection and 2.7 million people are newly infected yearly.[1] In 2006, an estimated 1.1 million people were living with HIV infection in the United States. About 21% of these patients remained undiagnosed.[2] In 2008, an estimated 56,300 people were newly infected with HIV in the United States.[3] As these data suggest, the epidemic clearly continues. As a result, emergency physicians worldwide face the challenge of caring for HIV-infected patients on a daily basis. Whether working in an inner city, suburban, or rural hospital, emergency physicians must maintain a basic knowledge of the medically complex and diverse disease processes that can affect this group of patients.

Before the mid 1990s, HIV-infected patients typically presented to the emergency department (ED) as young, previously healthy individuals suffering from the devastating effects of opportunistic infections and full-blown AIDS. There remained a relatively small number of illnesses that HIV-infected patients experienced and a limited knowledge of their therapies. Most opportunistic infections proved fatal within a short period. In stark contrast, recent years have shown the success of antiretroviral therapy (ART), as HIV-infected patients now present with a wide range of medical issues, many of them chronic in nature. ART has enabled these patients to live longer and experience fewer opportunistic complications while simultaneously uncovering a myriad of previously unknown comorbidities related to both the disease and its therapies. Research and clinical experience have revealed a wealth of information about the short- and long-term effects of the disease itself. From the elusive characteristics of acute HIV infection, to the more clinically obvious long-term sequelae of HIV, including nephropathy and coronary artery disease, HIV-infected patients have become a complex subset of the ED population. ARTs themselves have been shown to cause multiple complications such as insulin resistance, the metabolic syndrome, immune reconstitution inflammatory syndrome (IRIS), hepatic steatosis, and lactic acidosis. Given the multitude of recent advances and ongoing research in the area of HIV/AIDS, keeping up with this topic is no small task.

Emerg Med Clin N Am 28 (2010) xv–xvi
doi:10.1016/j.emc.2010.02.001
0733-8627/10/$ – see front matter © 2010 Elsevier Inc. All rights reserved.

emed.theclinics.com

This issue of *Emergency Medicine Clinics of North America* is the first one completely dedicated to the topic of HIV/AIDS. Our goal is to present the most recent information regarding HIV/AIDS with a focus on the details that are most valuable and necessary for the successful practice of emergency medicine. We have assembled a range of experts in the fields of infectious disease, dermatology, cardiology, immunology, neurology, pulmonology, and emergency care to create a comprehensive systems-based compilation of the key medical issues affecting the HIV-infected population. While reviewing some of the opportunistic infections that still afflict these patients, each article focuses primarily on the chronic illnesses and medication-related side effects that characterize the care of HIV-infected patients in the post-ART era. In addition to the systems-based articles, there are individual chapters specifically dedicated to topics of particular import to emergency physicians, including HIV testing in the ED, acute HIV, ART side effects, IRIS, and postexposure prophylaxis.

We would like to express our sincere appreciation to the authors who contributed their valuable time and effort to this issue. In addition, we would like to thank our families for their support and love. We hope that this issue will serve as a comprehensive resource for emergency physicians and others who continually to strive to provide optimal care to HIV-infected patients worldwide.

Mercedes Torres, MD
Department of Emergency Medicine
University of Maryland School of Medicine
110 South Paca Street, 6th Floor, Suite 200
Baltimore, MD 21201, USA

Rachel L. Chin, MD
Department of Emergency Medicine
San Francisco General Hospital
School of Medicine, University of California, San Francisco
1001 Potrero Avenue, 1E-21
San Francisco, CA 94110, USA

E-mail addresses:
mercedet@gmail.com (M. Torres)
Rachel.chin@emergency.ucsf.edu (R.L. Chin)

REFERENCES

1. UNAIDS. Report on the global AIDS epidemic. Available at: www.unaids.org; 2008. Accessed January 30, 2010.
2. CDC. HIV prevalence estimates—United States, 2006. MMWR Morb Mortal Wkly Rep 2008;57(39):1073–6.
3. Hall HI, Ruiguang S, Rhodes P, et al. Estimation of HIV incidence in the United States. JAMA 2008;300:520–9.

Head, Neck and Ophthalmologic Manifestations of HIV in the Emergency Department

Siamak Moayedi, MD

KEYWORDS

- Emergency medicine • Human immunodeficiency virus
- AIDS • Otolaryngology • Ophthalmology • HEENT

Nearly all patients with human immunodeficiency virus (HIV) and acquired immunodeficiency syndrome (AIDS) have some manifestation of their disease in the head and neck. The majority of these manifestations are due to opportunistic infections and malignancies as a direct result of immune suppression and the development of AIDS. On occasion some of these manifestations represent the initial signs of primary HIV infection. Since the introduction of potent antiretroviral therapies, the incidence of many of the diseases that are discussed in this article has decreased. However, knowledge of these diseases will allow the emergency physician to recognize new diagnoses, treatment failures, and progression of HIV/AIDS. In some cases, prompt diagnosis and therapy will lead to preservation of function and prevention of significant morbidity.

PATHOLOGY OF THE HEAD AND NECK
Oral Candidiasis

Despite the numerous species of yeast, *Candida albicans* is by far the most common pathogen responsible for oral candidiasis. There are 3 different ways that oral *Candida* infections can be manifested: pseudomembranous form, atrophic form, and angular cheilitis. The predominant form is thrush, a pseudomembranous eruption presenting as white plaques that can occur on virtually any mucus membrane within the oral cavity. For the most part, thrush is asymptomatic, but heavy infestation can give a sense of cotton and dryness in the mouth along with loss of taste. The visualized

Department of Emergency Medicine, University of Maryland, School of Medicine, 110 South Paca Street, Sixth Floor, Suite 200, Baltimore, MD 21201, USA
E-mail address: Smoay001@yahoo.com

Emerg Med Clin N Am 28 (2010) 265–271
doi:10.1016/j.emc.2010.01.006
0733-8627/10/$ – see front matter © 2010 Elsevier Inc. All rights reserved.

plaques can be wiped or scraped off. A less common, but painful manifestation of oral candidiasis is the atrophic form, which manifests as flat, red, painful ulcerations and represents a more invasive infection. Angular cheilitis is a painful, flaking, fissuring, and red irritation of the angles of the lips. The diagnosis is often made by visual inspection; however, microscopic evaluation can be performed after application of potassium hydroxide yields pseudohyphae and budding yeast cells. Treatment of mild to moderate cases involves topical antifungal suspensions such as nystatin. More aggressive forms will require oral systemic antifungals such as fluconazole. When oral candidiasis is associated with odynophagia, dysphagia, and retrosternal pain, the diagnosis of esophageal candidiasis must be entertained. This entity qualifies as an AIDS-defining illness.

Oral Hairy Leukoplakia

Oral hairy leukoplakia can be confused with oral candidiasis. Oral hairy leukoplakia represents hypertrophy of the tongue's squamous epithelium as a consequence of infection with the Epstein-Barr virus. The lateral aspects of the tongue are predominantly covered with a white, thick, irregular, and painless layer. Other parts of the tongue, buccal mucosa, and palate can also be involved. Unlike thrush, the lesions cannot be scraped off. The diagnosis, if in question, can be confirmed histologically. This diagnosis is a very sensitive clinical indicator of AIDS as it is rarely seen in patients with other immunodeficiencies.[1] Fortunately, oral hairy leukoplakia is not considered to be a premalignant lesion. Treatment is seldom required as the process is often asymptomatic, and tends to spontaneously resolve and recur.[1]

Kaposi Sarcoma

Kaposi sarcoma is the most common AIDS-related oral malignancy and is considered an AIDS-defining illness. The pathogenesis is related to the sexually transmitted human herpes virus 8.[2] This malignancy tends to occur predominantly in men who have sex with men.[3] The lesions progress from macular patches with blue color to dark raised plaques that may ulcerate. Although cutaneous lesions are common, oral involvement occurs in one-third of patients and in 15% of cases represents the initial site of malignancy.[4] When the nasal mucosa is involved, patients can present with the sensation of nasal obstruction or epistaxis.[5]

Gingivitis and Periodontal Disease

Linear gingival erythema (previously called HIV-gingivitis) is characterized by a brightly inflamed and well-delineated area of redness on the border of the gingiva. This condition is painful, and susceptible to bleeding with minor trauma. The etiology is multifactorial and includes gram-negative anaerobes, enteric species, and yeast. The extreme version of this condition is termed necrotizing periodontal disease (typically occurring in patients with CD4 counts <400 cells/mm^3), which is caused by similar organisms often in conjunction with a concurrent herpes virus infection.[6] Necrotizing periodontal disease is characterized by rapid tissue destruction and sloughing, with subsequent periodontal detachment due to alveolar bone necrosis.[7] The patient often presents to the emergency department with severe mouth pain, bleeding, and halitosis. Also known as "trench mouth," this disease is not limited to HIV-infected patients, and has been additionally linked to malnutrition and other forms of impaired immune response.[7] Treatment involves pain control, antibiotic therapy, chlorhexidine gluconate mouth rinses, and close follow-up by the periodontist.

Oral Ulcerations

HIV-infected and AIDS patients are more susceptible to oral viral infections and vesicular lesions. Recurrent aphthus ulcers occur in up to 13% of HIV-infected patients, especially once the CD4 count decreases to less than 100 cells/mm^3.[8] There are many viruses capable of producing these painful lesions, including cytomegalovirus (CMV) and herpes simplex virus reactivation. HIV itself can cause ulcerations in the early stages of infection. In general, these lesions tend to be present for a more prolonged period of time. Eruptions tend to be more severe and are at higher risk of complication with superinfection.

Acute HIV Infection

Recognition of acute HIV infection can lead to prevention of disease spread and progress. Unfortunately, the viral syndrome associated with acute HIV infection can be challenging to distinguish from other infections. Although the incubation period varies, within 2 to 4 weeks of HIV transmission the patient typically develops fever, sore throat, nausea, dry cough, and other flu-like symptoms.[9] One of the most distinguishing features of acute HIV infection is the presence of painful, shallow, well-demarcated ulcers on the mouth, anus, or penis. The location of the ulcers is thought to be the mucus membrane where HIV transmission occurred.[9] This early period of acute HIV infection is a time of high viral load and infectivity, while the patient is often unaware that they have contracted the virus. This situation is complicated by the fact that seroconversion typically occurs within 4 to 10 weeks after exposure (>95% after 6 months), therefore traditional HIV testing may not initially reveal the diagnosis.[10] A viral load can assist with diagnosis at this early stage.[11]

Lymphadenopathy

Persistent generalized lymphadenopathy is found in up to 11% of patients with early HIV infection.[12] In general, these enlarged lymph nodes occur within 10 months of seroconversion. The nodes are typically nontender, measure less than 5 mm, and occur most commonly in the posterior cervical chain with respect to the head and neck area.[9] More significant causes of lymphadenopathy occur with advancing immunosuppression, and may represent the diagnosis of tuberculosis, lymphoma, histoplasmosis, or other diseases characteristic of immunocompromise.[5]

Parotid Enlargement

An early persistent clue to HIV infection is the presence of unilateral or bilateral, mildly tender, soft parotid masses. Fine-needle aspiration of fluid within a parotid mass can be submitted to pathology. The pathologic diagnosis of a benign lymphoepithelial cyst is highly specific to HIV infection.[13] These cysts enlarge within the parotid glands bilaterally as a consequence of intraparotid lymph node hyperplasia.[5] These benign cysts are strongly associated with the generalized lymphadenopathy that occurs early in the course of HIV infection.[13] Less common solid masses of the parotid glands have a 40% chance of being malignant.[14] HIV-associated parotid malignancies include lymphoma and Kaposi sarcoma.

Sinusitis

Recurrent sinusitis occurs more frequently in HIV-infected patients. The cause is thought to be related to a host of factors including decreased immune response, increased allergic response, and decreased mucociliary clearance.[15] During acute HIV, the presenting signs and symptoms of sinusitis are similar to immunocompetent patients. However, with progression to AIDS, patients develop the potential for invasive fungal sinusitis. This rapidly progressive infection can invade structures posterior to the sinuses and result in significant morbidity and mortality. The most common fungi species responsible for this infection include *Mucor, Rhizopus*, and *Aspergillus*.[15] Pain out of proportion to external physical examination, often manifested as excruciating pain at the site of invasion, may be the only clue to the presence of invasive fungal sinusitis.[16] Immediate otolaryngology consultation for surgical debridement and prompt institution of systemic antifungal medication is the mainstay of therapy.

Seborrheic Dermatitis

Seborrheic dermatitis is an inflammatory condition related to overgrowth of fungal skin flora and an overproduction of skin cells and natural oils. The symptoms include pruritic, erythematous, greasy, and scaly patches on the head, eyebrows, and other parts of the body rich with oil ducts. Extensive seborrheic dermatitis has been described with advancing HIV disease. Up to 80% of AIDS patients and 40% of HIV patients have some degree of this dermatitis.[17] Seborrheic dermatitis in this population is more severe and unfortunately often refractory to treatment.[17] Furthermore, due to the intense pruritus and inflammatory process, the affected skin is at increased risk for superinfection with invasive bacteria. The possibility of HIV infection should be considered in patients presenting with new onset of severe seborrheic dermatitis.

Hearing Loss

Ototoxic antiretroviral medications include azidothymidine, dideoxyinosine, and dideoxycytidine. Other treatment-related medications that can impact hearing include trimethoprim-sulfamethoxazole and acyclovir.[5] As with most other infections, HIV-infected patients are also at higher risk of bacterial and fungal infections both pre- and post-tympanic membrane, which can lead to hearing loss. Herpes zoster virus reactivation can cause a polyneuropathy involving multiple cranial nerves and can lead to Ramsey-Hunt syndrome, clinically characterized by ear pain, vesicles in the auditory canal, hearing loss, facial nerve paralysis, and vertigo. Finally, neoplasms such as lymphoma and Kaposi sarcoma can cause hearing loss.

Molluscum Contagiosum

Caused by a poxvirus, molluscum contagiosum occurs in up to 13% of AIDS patients.[18] Typically a minor dermal disease of young children, the increase of molluscum infections in adults is attributed to the prevalence of AIDS.[19] Molluscum is spread by skin to skin contact and can occur anywhere on the body. The lesions are translucent, firm, centrally umbilicated papules that can occur on the face, neck, scalp, eyelids, and conjunctiva. AIDS patients' lesions can persist chronically, appearing more numerous and disfiguring, whereas eruptions in immunocompetent patients are self-limited.

PATHOLOGY OF THE EYES

Ophthalmic disease affects up to 80% of patients with HIV infection at some time during the natural history of their infection.[20] There are many ways that HIV infection can involve the eyes. From the perspective of emergency medicine, these can be categorized into 2 areas. First, the retina is affected by opportunistic infections such as cytomegalovirus or vasculopathy as a direct result of HIV infection. Second, the ocular surface can be involved with infections such as herpes zoster virus.

CMV Retinitis

CMV is a double-stranded DNA virus in the herpes family. CMV retinitis is the most common ophthalmologic complication of AIDS. Furthermore, retinitis is the most common clinical presentation of CMV infection. Before AIDS, there were very few described cases of CMV retinitis in the medical literature. Before the introduction of potent antiretroviral therapy (ART), 30% of AIDS patients would develop CMV retinitis.[21] Significant immunosuppression needs to occur (CD4 count <50 cells/mm³) for CMV to become clinically significant. CMV reaches the retina through the blood stream and starts as a single lesion, advancing outward. Depending on the location and size of the lesion within the retina, patients present with blurred vision, the sensation of seeing floaters, and visual scotomas. On fundoscopic examination, early retinitis is seen as small white perivascular infiltrates.[22] With disease progression, hemorrhagic necrotizing retinitis with clusters of small white retinal infiltrates in the periphery is visualized.[22] As the necrosis advances across the retina, tears can develop and lead to retinal detachment. Blindness can occur within 4 to 6 months of infection.[22] CMV retinitis is responsible for 40% of vision loss in AIDS patients.[21] Treatment of CMV retinitis includes starting ART and treating the CMV infection. Choice of anti-CMV medication depends on the location and extent of the infection, and is deferred to the ophthalmologist. Valganciclovir typically is recommended, given its high bioavailability when taken in the oral form.[21] Several other agents can be given intravenously or even injected or implanted in the vitreous of the affected eye. Most importantly, treatment must continue indefinitely until the immunodeficiency resolves.

CMV Immune Recovery Uveitis

Immune recovery uveitis is a reaction to CMV antigens within the eye as a result of immune recovery after initiation of ART.[21] Within weeks of starting treatment, up to 15.5% of patients with CMV retinitis will experience intense eye pain, photophobia, decreased visual acuity, and floaters.[23] Slit lamp and fundoscopic examination will reveal an intense inflammatory reaction involving the anterior chamber, vitreous body, and retina. In some patients, this inflammatory reaction will lead to macular edema or cataract formation, causing significant vision loss.[21] Treatment involves prompt ophthalmology referral along with antivirals for CMV and temporary discontinuation of ART.

HIV Retinopathy

There is an increased prevalence of vision abnormalities including abnormal color vision, visual field deficits, and light contrast perception in HIV-infected patients.[24] These visual abnormalities increase with progression to AIDS. On fundoscopic examination, cotton-wool spots and retinal hemorrhages are clues to the presence of HIV retinopathy. Indeed, cotton-wool spots (also seen in diabetic retinopathy) represent the most common ophthalmologic finding in AIDS.[25] The process by which HIV infection leads to retinopathy is not well understood. However, a microvasculopathy resulting in the narrowing of retinal capillaries has been reported in autopsies of AIDS patients.[21] It is thought that this microvasculopathy leads to the destruction of both retinal and optic nerves. Cotton-wool spots represent a risk factor for CMV retinitis as an area that can facilitate transmission of CMV-infected leukocytes across vessel walls.[21]

Herpes Zoster Ophthalmicus

HIV-infected patients have a higher rate of ocular complication with herpes zoster infection. If zoster lesions involve the tip of the nose (Hutchinson sign), ophthalmologic evaluation is necessary. The nasociliary branch of cranial nerve 5 (first division) innervates both the tip of the nose and the surface of the eye.[5] Early diagnosis is critical in order to prevent corneal involvement and potential loss of vision. Treatment involves antibiotics targeting the herpes zoster virus and topical steroid drops to reduce the inflammatory response.

In addition to affecting the cornea, the retina can be involved, leading to zoster retinitis. This retinal infection can occur concurrent with, after, or even in the absence of any other cutaneous zoster lesions.[26] The condition is frequently bilateral, suggesting a hematogenous route of dissemination.[26] The most significant complications of retinal involvement are acute retinal necrosis and retinal detachment, ultimately causing blindness.

SUMMARY

Emergency physicians are uniquely positioned to detect manifestations of HIV disease in the head and neck region. Awareness of the myriad of opportunistic infections and malignancies that involve the head, neck, and eyes is paramount to their diagnosis and treatment. In many cases, the presence of such diseases is a clue to the diagnosis of HIV infection or progression to AIDS. Many of these infections, if not detected early, will lead to significant morbidity and mortality.

REFERENCES

1. Triantos D, Porter SR, Scully C, et al. Oral hairy leukoplakia: clinicopathologic features, pathogenesis, diagnosis, and clinical significance. Clin Infect Dis 1997;25(6):1392–6.
2. Moore PS, Chang Y. Detection of herpesvirus-like DNA sequences in Kaposi's sarcoma in patients with and without HIV infection. N Engl J Med 1995;332(18): 1181–5.
3. Beral V, Peterman TA, Berkelman RL, et al. Kaposi's sarcoma among persons with AIDS: a sexually transmitted infection? Lancet 1990;335(8682):123–8.
4. Nichols CM, Flaitz CM, Hick MJ. Treating Kaposi's lesions in the HIV-infected patient. J Am Dent Assoc 1993;124(11):78–84.
5. Gurney TA, Murr AH. Otolaryngologic manifestations of human immunodeficiency virus infection. Otolaryngol Clin North Am 2003;36:607–24.
6. Slots J. Herpesvirus, the missing link between gingivitis and periodontitis? J Int Acad Periodontol 2004;6(4):113–9.
7. Mosca NG, Hathorn AR. HIV-positive patients: dental management considerations. Dent Clin North Am 2006;50(4):635–57.
8. Reichart PA. Oral ulcerations in HIV infection. Oral Dis 1997;3(Suppl 1):S180–2.
9. Gaines H, von Sydow M, Pehrson PO, et al. Clinical picture of primary HIV infection presenting as a glandular-fever-like illness. BMJ 1988;297(6660):1363–8.
10. Coutlee F, Olivier C, Cassol S, et al. Absence of prolonged immunosilent infection with human immunodeficiency virus in individuals with high-risk behaviors. Am J Med 1994;96(1):42–8.
11. Daar ES, Little S, Pitt J, et al. Diagnosis of primary HIV-1 infection. Los Angeles County Primary HIV Infection Recruitment Network. Ann Intern Med 2001; 134(1):25–9.
12. Lang W, Anderson RE, Perkins H, et al. Clinical, immunologic and serologic findings in men at risk for acquired immunodeficiency syndrome: the San Francisco Men's Health Study. JAMA 1992;25:326–30.
13. Som PM, Brandwein MS, Silvers A. Nodal inclusion cysts of the parotid gland and parapharyngeal space: a discussion of lymphoepithelial, AIDS-related parotid

and brachial cysts, cystic Warthin's tumors and cysts in Sjögren's syndrome. Laryngoscope 1995;105:1122–8.

14. Huang RD, Pearlman S, Friedman WH, et al. Benign cystic vs. solids lesions of the parotid gland in HIV patients. Head Neck 1991;13:522–7.

15. Tami TA. The management of sinusitis in patients infected with the human immunodeficiency virus. Ear Nose Throat J 1995;74(5):360–3.

16. Hunt SM, Miyamoto RC, Cornelius RS, et al. Invasive fungal sinusitis in the acquired immunodeficiency syndrome. Otolaryngol Clin North Am 2000;33(2): 335–47.

17. Mathes BM, Douglass MC. Seborrheic dermatitis in patients with acquired immunodeficiency syndrome. J Am Acad Dermatol 1985;13(6):947–51.

18. Reisacher WR, Finn DG, Stern J, et al. Manifestations of AIDS in the head and neck. South Med J 1999;92(7):684–97.

19. Koopman RJ, van Merrienboer FC, Vreden SG, et al. Molluscum contagiosum; a marker for advanced HIV infection. Br J Dermatol 1992;126:528.

20. Cunningham ET, Margolis TP. Ocular manifestations of HIV infection. N Engl J Med 1998;339:236–44.

21. Holland GN. AIDS and ophthalmology: the first quarter century. Am J Ophthalmol 2008;145:397–408.

22. See RF, Rao NA. Cytomegalovirus retinitis in the era of combined highly active antiretroviral therapy. Ophthalmol Clin North Am 2002;15:529–36.

23. Jabs DA, Van Natta ML, Kempen JH, et al. Characteristics of patients with cytomegalovirus retinitis in the era of highly active antiretroviral therapy. Am J Ophthalmol 2002;133(1):48–61.

24. Freeman WR, van Natta ML, Jabs DA, et al. Vision function in HIV-infected individuals without retinitis: report of the Studies of Ocular Complications of AIDS Research Group. Am J Ophthalmol 2008;145:453–62.

25. Pepose JS, Holland GN, Nestor M, et al. Acquired immune deficiency syndrome: pathogenic mechanisms of ocular disease. Ophthalmology 1985;92:472–84.

26. Glesby MJ, Moore RD, Chaisson RE. Clinical spectrum of herpes zoster in adults infected with human immunodeficiency virus. Clin Infect Dis 1995;21(2):311–5.

Cardiac Emergencies in Patients with HIV

Rakesh K. Mishra, MD

KEYWORDS

- HIV • Cardiovascular disease • Acute coronary syndrome
- Pericardial effusion • Cardiomyopathy

The topic of cardiovascular disease in patients infected with human immunodeficiency virus (HIV) has changed significantly since the introduction of antiretroviral therapy (ART). In the early years of the HIV epidemic, the principal cardiovascular manifestations of HIV were dilated cardiomyopathy, pericardial disease, pulmonary hypertension, and neoplastic involvement of the heart. ART has been revolutionary in the care of HIV patients, significantly reducing the incidence of opportunistic infections and, thereby, prolonging life.[1] However, ART can be associated with significant metabolic abnormalities including insulin resistance, lipid abnormalities such as decreased high-density lipoproteins (HDL) and increased triglycerides, and fat redistribution syndromes with a general loss of peripheral fat and intraabdominal fat accumulation.[2] Therefore, it is not surprising that, as the incidence of dilated cardiomyopathy and pericardial disease has decreased in the ART era, the incidence of cardiovascular disease has increased. The prolongation of life with ART, the increasing duration of exposure to antiretroviral agents throughout a patient's lifetime, and HIV infection itself may all be factors in the increasing incidence and prevalence of cardiovascular disease in patients infected with HIV.

The aspects of cardiovascular disease in the patient infected with HIV that are of particular relevance to the emergency physician, including coronary artery disease (CAD) and acute coronary syndromes, pericardial disease, and dilated cardiomyopathy are discussed in this review.

RISK OF CAD

Although some controversy still remains, there seems to be an increased rate of coronary events in patients infected with HIV. Although side effects of ART may contribute to some of the increased rate of CAD in patients infected with HIV,[3–11] ongoing viral replication in untreated HIV infection is also a likely factor in the development of CAD.[12] The data on the possible role of ART in the increased risk of cardiovascular

Dr Rakesh K. Mishra is on the speakers' bureau of GlaxoSmithKline, Inc.
Berkeley Cardiovascular Medical Group, 2450 Ashby Avenue, Berkeley, CA 94705, USA
E-mail address: rmishrasf@yahoo.com

Emerg Med Clin N Am 28 (2010) 273–282
doi:10.1016/j.emc.2010.01.005
0733-8627/10/$ – see front matter © 2010 Elsevier Inc. All rights reserved.

emed.theclinics.com

disease in patients infected with HIV and the contribution of HIV itself is reviewed in **Table 1**.

HIV, ART and Metabolic Syndromes

HIV and ART are both associated with lipid derangements and metabolic abnormalities that may contribute to the development of CAD. Riddler and colleagues[13] reported that, in 50 patients in the Multicenter AIDS Cohort Study for whom preinfection sera were available, levels of total cholesterol, low-density lipoprotein (LDL) and HDL decreased after HIV infection by 22 mg/dL, 12 mg/dL, and 30 mg/dL, respectively. After initiation of ART, total and LDL cholesterol returned to preinfection levels but HDL levels remained decreased. Among the various components of ART, protease inhibitors (PIs) are associated with hyperlipidemia, specifically increased total and LDL cholesterol levels, and insulin resistance.[14] Insulin resistance precedes the lipodystrophy, an HIV-associated fat redistribution from peripheral to central and visceral sites, which affects 20% to 35% of patients after 1 to 2 years of ART.[15,16] In addition to insulin resistance, lipodystrophy in patients infected with HIV is associated with other components of the metabolic syndrome, such as increased triglyceride levels, low HDL, and hypertension.[17,18] This abnormal distribution of fat is not ameliorated by limiting caloric intake but may respond to exercise in combination with metformin.[19] These metabolic derangements, encompassing lipid abnormalities, fat redistribution, and insulin resistance, are all significant risk factors for CAD.

ART and its Role in CAD

The HIV Outpatient Study (HOPS), a large prospective observational study, found an increase in the incidence of myocardial infarction (MI) after the introduction of PIs in 1996 (see **Table 1**).[3] The Data Collection on Adverse Events of Anti-HIV Drugs (D:A:D) Study Group, another large prospective observational study, also showed that the incidence of MI increased with increasing exposure to combination ART (P for trend <0.001). In a follow-up study, the adjusted relative risk of MI was 1.16 (95% CI 1.10–1.23) per year of exposure to PI.[9]

In yet another study from the same cohort, exposure within the preceding 6 months to 2 nucleoside reverse transcriptase inhibitors (NRTIs), abacavir and didanosine, was associated with an increased risk of MI.[11] In the French Hospital Database, there were 60 MIs in 34,976 HIV patients followed for a median period of 33 months.[6] In multivariate analysis, older age and exposure to PIs (specifically lopinavir/ritonavir and fosamprenavir/ritonavir in multivariate analyses) were significant predictors of MI.

Contrary to the studies discussed earlier, 2 studies have failed to show an association with either HIV or ART (whether PIs or NRTIs) and the risk of MI.[4,5] Klein and colleagues[4] compared 4159 men infected with HIV, aged 35 to 64 years, enrolled in the Kaiser Permanente Medical Care Program of Northern California with 39,877 age-matched controls not infected with HIV. The overall coronary heart disease (CHD) rate among patients infected with HIV was significantly greater than that of the controls (6.5 vs 3.8 events per 1000 person-years; P = .003). The age-adjusted CHD and MI hospitalization rates were not significantly different before and after PIs (6.2 vs 6.7 events per 1000 person-years) or before and after the initiation of ART (5.7 vs 6.7 events per 1000 person-years).

A retrospective study of 36,766 patients infected with HIV in the Veterans Affairs (VA) system followed for a mean period of 40 months found no relation between the use of nucleoside analogs, PIs, or non-NRTIs and the risk of cardiovascular or cerebrovascular events.[5] Between 1995 and 2001, the rate of admissions for cardiovascular or cerebrovascular disease decreased from 1.7 to 0.9 per 100 patient-years and the

Table 1
HIV, HAART, and cardiovascular disease

Study	Patients (n)	Age (y)	Male (%)	Follow-up	Events	Results
VA study	36,766	n.s.	98.1	40 months	1207 CHD admissions	No association of ART and CHD
HOPS	5672	42.6 (mean)	82	3.1 years	21 MIs	Increased risk of MI with PI exposure
DAD study group	23,437	39 (median)	75.9	4.5 years (median)	345 MIs	Increased risk of MI with PI exposure
French hospital	34,976		100	2.5 years	66 MIs	Increased risk of MI with PI exposure
Kaiser study	4159	43.6 (mean)	100	4.1 years (median)	72 CHD hospitalizations, including 47 MIs	No association of ART with CHD
DAD study group	33,447	49 (median)	92	5.1 years (median)	517 MIs	Increased risk of MI with recent exposure to abacavir or didanosine

Abbreviations: CHD, coronary heart disease; MI, myocardial infarction; n, number; n.s., not specified; PI, protease inhibitor.
Data from Refs.[3–7,11]

rate of death from any cause decreased from 21.3 to 5.9 deaths per 100 patient-years. The reasons for the discrepancy between the results of these 2 studies and the others remain unclear but perhaps reflect different study designs based on ecological-level data versus individual-level data.[20]

Ongoing Viral Replication as a Risk Factor for CAD

The Strategies for Management of Antiretroviral Therapy (SMART) trial provided some insight into the possible mechanism of why cardiovascular events have increased in the ART era.[12] This study randomized 5472 individuals who were HIV-positive with CD4 counts higher than 350 cells/mm^3 on therapy to a management strategy of staying on continuous ART versus intermittent use of ART depending on their CD4 counts. Participants in the latter arm would stop taking ARTs when their CD4 cell count reached greater than 350 cells/mm^3 and restart therapy once the CD4 count reached 250 cells/mm^3 or less. The results of the trial showed that more patients in the interrupted therapy arm suffered serious HIV-related events, which was not unexpected. However, surprisingly, patients in the discontinuous therapy arm had a 1.5-fold (95% CI 1.0–2.2) greater risk of severe complications not related to HIV such as nonfatal cardiovascular events (RR 1.5 with 95% 1.0–2.5).

The association between uncontrolled viral replication and complications not related to AIDS, such as cardiovascular disease and non-AIDS malignancies, has now been verified in several cohort settings.[21] This, combined with the dramatic decrease in overall mortality in the HIV-infected population on ART, suggests that any minor contributions that certain PIs or NRTIs may make to the risk of CAD are likely outweighed by the risk of ongoing viral replication in patients with HIV infection, thus strengthening the case for initiating and maintaining patients on virologically suppressive ART regimens.

CLINICAL AND ANGIOGRAPHIC FINDINGS IN PATIENTS INFECTED WITH HIV WITH ACUTE CORONARY SYNDROME

The typical HIV-infected patient presenting with acute coronary syndrome (ACS) is a man in his mid to late 40s. The most common presentation is an acute MI, most often with ST segment elevation. Coronary anatomy seems to be variable, with some studies showing a higher prevalence of single-vessel disease and others showing a higher prevalence of 2- and 3-vessel disease than controls not infected with HIV.

Many case series of patients infected with HIV presenting with ACS have now been published (**Table 2**).[22–27] Escaut and colleagues[22] followed a cohort of 840 patients infected with HIV and observed coronary events in 17 patients in a 7-year period. Fifteen of these patients were men and individuals with coronary events were slightly older than the general cohort (45.6 ± 5.89 vs 43 ± 9.4 years; P = .03). Eleven patients presented with acute MIs, all with ST segment elevation; 3 presented with unstable angina, and 3 with angina pectoris. All patients underwent coronary angiography, which revealed single-vessel disease in about half the patients.

Mehta and colleagues[23] performed a comprehensive search of the literature for cases of CAD associated with HIV. Of the 129 cases identified, the mean age was 42.3 ± 10.2 years and 91% were male. Most patients (77%) presented with an acute MI and the rest presented with unstable angina. In the 76 patients for whom angiographic data were available, 36 (47%) had 3-vessel disease, 14 (18%) had 2-vessel disease, and 26 (35%) had single-vessel disease.

In a series of 51 patients with HIV and ACS by Ambrose and colleagues,[24] 92% were male and the mean age was 48 ± 9 years. Thirty-four patients (67%) presented with an

Table 2
Acute MI and PCI in patients infected with HIV

Study	Patients (n)	Men (n)	Age (y)	Acute MI (n)	3-Vessel Disease (n)	PCI (n)	Stents (n)	Follow-up (mo)	Restenosis (n)
Escaut et al[22]	17	15	45 ± 6	11	5	17	11	36	5
Ambrose et al[24]	51	47	48 ± 9	34	9	25	21	n.s.	n.s.
Matetzky et al[28]	24	21	47 ± 9	24	n.s.	17	n.s.	14.7	6
Hsue et al[25]	68	61	50 ± 8	37	n.s.	29	22	n.s.	15
Boccara et al[27]	20	19	44 ± 8	20	5	9	9	38	0

Abbreviations: n, number; n.s., not specified.

acute MI, including 16 patients (31%) with non-ST elevation MI (NSTEMI), and 17 patients (33%) presented with unstable angina. In the 45 patients who underwent coronary angiography, 5 (11%) had no obstructive CAD, 21 (47%) had single-vessel disease, 10 (22%) had 2-vessel disease, and 9 (20%) had 3-vessel disease.

Matetzky and colleagues[28] reported on a series of 24 consecutive patients infected with HIV admitted with acute MI. The mean age was 47 ± 9 years and 88% were male. Fourteen patients (58%) presented with STEMI and the rest (10 patients, 42%) had NSTEMIs. Twenty-one patients underwent coronary angiography, with 16 (76%) having multivessel CAD.

Hsue and colleagues[25] published a series of 68 patients infected with HIV and 68 randomly selected patients admitted with ACS to an urban hospital. The patients infected with HIV with ACS were younger, with a male predominance. More patients infected with HIV presented with unstable angina (31/68 vs 19/68; $P<.001$) than controls not infected with HIV. The patients infected with HIV presenting with unstable angina and NSTEMI had a lower thrombolysis in MI (TIMI) risk score. There was no significant difference between the patients infected with HIV and the control group in total numbers of STEMI (20/68 vs 24/68; $P = .46$) and NSTEMI (17/68 vs 25/68; $P = .14$). Fifty-six of the patients infected with HIV and 61 of the control group underwent coronary angiography. The control group had more extensive CAD than the patients infected with HIV.

In another series of 20 patients infected with HIV with ACS reported by Boccara and colleagues,[27] the mean age was 44 ± 8 years and 95% were men. Fifteen presented with STEMI (8 anterior, 5 inferior, and 2 lateral) and 5 with NSTEMI. All patients underwent coronary angiography, which revealed single-vessel disease in 12 patients (60%), 2-vessel disease in 2 patients (10%), 3-vessel disease in 5 patients (25%), normal coronary arteries in 1 patient (5%), and left ventricular thrombus in 2 patients (10%).

These observational studies suggest that the patient infected with HIV presenting with ACS is younger and more likely to present with acute MI than a person who is HIV-negative and may have single- or multivessel CAD.

EFFECTIVENESS OF CORONARY REVASCULARIZATION

Percutaneous coronary intervention (PCI) with and without stenting and coronary artery bypass grafting (CABG) are feasible in the setting of ACS,[22–29] regardless of

HIV infection status (see **Table 2**). Of the 14 patients infected with HIV presenting with ACS in the series by Escaut and colleagues,[22] 11 underwent coronary angioplasty with stenting. At 12 months after PCI, restenosis occurred in 5 of the 11 patients. Among the 45 patients who underwent coronary angiography in the series by Ambrose and colleagues,[24] 25 patients underwent PCI with 21 receiving stents, 9 underwent CABG, 6 were treated medically, and 5 had no significant CAD. In-hospital revascularization mortality was limited to 1 patient who underwent CABG (1 out of 34; 3%). There were no in-hospital deaths in the PCI group. In the series by Matetzky and colleagues,[28] 21 of the 24 patients underwent coronary angiography during the index hospitalization. Of the 14 patients presenting with STEMI, 12 underwent immediate PCI. Overall, 17 patients underwent PCI and 3 patients had CABG. There were no deaths or re-infarctions during the in-hospital period. During a period of 14.7 ± 8.0 months, 14 patients were followed up after successful PCI. Six of these patients (43%) required target vessel revascularization for recurrent ischemia and restenosis. In the study by Hsue and colleagues,[25] 29 patients infected with HIV and 21 controls underwent PCI, and 22 patients infected with HIV and 11 controls received stents. More patients in the control group were referred for CABG (16 vs 6; $P = .032$); 15 patients infected with HIV and 3 controls subsequently developed restenosis (52% vs 14%; $P = .006$). Among those who received stents, 11 of the 22 patients infected with HIV and 2 of the 11 controls developed restenosis (50% vs 18%; $P = .078$). Among the 20 patients infected with HIV presenting with ACS reported by Boccara and colleagues,[27] 4 patients were treated with thrombolysis, 2 had primary coronary angioplasty with stenting, and 7 had secondary coronary angioplasty with stenting (including 2 who had had primary thrombolysis), guided by the result of stress testing. There were no in-hospital deaths and, at a mean follow-up of 38 ± 15 months, no patients who initially had PCI needed target vessel revascularization. In another study of Boccara and colleagues[29] comparing immediate results and long-term prognosis in patients infected with HIV undergoing PCI with controls, clinical restenosis at follow-up was not significantly different between those infected with HIV and those who were not(14% vs 16%; $P = .78$).

CABG seems to be a feasible technique for revascularization in patients infected with HIV. Boccara and colleagues[30] compared 27 consecutive patients infected with HIV and 54 controls without HIV infection undergoing CABG. At 30 days, both groups had identical rates of major adverse cardiovascular events (MACE). At a median follow-up of 41 months, there was a higher rate of MACE in the HIV-infected group versus controls (11, 42% vs 13, 25%; $P = .03$), mostly because of the need for repeat revascularization using PCI of the native coronary arteries but not of the grafts.

These studies suggest that PCI with and without stenting is a safe and effective therapy in patients infected with HIV presenting with ACS. Although the in-hospital mortality after PCI is low, some studies do suggest a higher rate of restenosis in patients infected with HIV. In addition, CABG is a safe and feasible procedure in patients infected with HIV with multivessel CAD, with an unremarkable postoperative outcome but an increased rate of repeat revascularization of the native coronary arteries in the long-term.

SHORT- AND LONG-TERM PROGNOSIS AFTER ACS AND PCI

Short-term prognosis is good for patients infected with HIV with ACS, with generally low in-hospital mortality. Although long-term event-free survival is also quite good, there does seem to be a relatively higher incidence of recurrent ischemic events in patients infected with HIV compared with those without HIV infection.

In-hospital mortality ranged from 0% to 8% in earlier studies,[22,24,27,28] with later reports showing lower in-hospital mortality rates. In the series by Escaut and colleagues,[22] 14 of the 17 patients were alive at a mean follow-up of 36 months. During a follow-up of 14.7 ± 8.0 months, Matetzky and colleagues[28] reported no deaths in the 24 HIV patients who had presented with acute MI. However, there was a high incidence of reinfarction (4 [20%]) and rehospitalization for recurrent coronary events (9 [45%]). In the first series by Boccara and colleagues,[27] 10 of 20 patients had 18 recurrent cardiovascular events at a follow-up of 38 ± 15 months. There was 1 cardiovascular death as a result of cardiogenic shock and 7 episodes of recurrent myocardial ischemia in 4 patients.

In the second larger study by Boccara and colleagues[29] comparing 50 patients with HIV and 50 without HIV undergoing PCI for STEMI, NSTEMI, unstable angina, and stable angina pectoris, the in-hospital course was uneventful in both groups, including no acute stent thromboses. At a mean follow-up of 625 days, there were no deaths in either group. Both groups had similar low rates of clinical restenosis including the need for target vessel revascularization (14% in HIV-positive vs 16% in HIV-negative; $P = .78$), similar event-free survival rates (80% in HIV-positive vs 84% in HIV-negative; $P = .64$), and occurrence of MI (8% in HIV-positive vs 0% in HIV-negative; $P = .12$).

These studies suggest reasonably good short- and long-term prognosis for patients infected with HIV with ACS, with a relatively higher incidence of recurrent ischemic events.

PERICARDIAL DISEASE IN HIV

In the pre-ART era, the incidence of pericardial effusion in patients infected with HIV was 11% per year.[31] A male predominance in the development of pericardial effusions has been reported.[32] Dyspnea and edema were common presenting symptoms, whereas chest pain was uncommon.[32] Most of the effusions were small with a lower prevalence of moderate to large pericardial effusions.[31–33] Variables associated with moderate to large pericardial effusions were congestive heart failure, Kaposi sarcoma, tuberculosis, and pulmonary infections of all causes.[33] Tamponade requiring emergent pericardiocentesis was rare, as was acute pericarditis, even in the pre-ART era.[31,33] The development of a pericardial effusion is a poor prognostic marker in patients with HIV.[31] Pericardiocentesis is currently recommended only in large symptomatic effusions, for diagnostic evaluation of systemic illness, or for the management of acute cardiac tamponade.[34] The prevalence of pericardial effusions has declined dramatically, however, since the introduction of ART (13.5%–3.4%).[35]

DILATED CARDIOMYOPATHY IN HIV

Dilated cardiomyopathy was a common cardiac complication of HIV infection in the pre-ART era with a prevalence of 10% to 30%.[36] Congestive heart failure associated with myocardial dysfunction was present in approximately 2% of patients infected with HIV[37] in a report from 1993. Patients infected with HIV with dilated cardiomyopathy had a much lower survival rate than those without (mean 101 days, 95% CI 42–146 vs 472 days, 95% 383–560).[38] Although cardiotropic viral infection was demonstrated by myocardial biopsy in almost all cases of HIV-related dilated cardiomyopathy, other causes, such as nutritional deficiencies, autonomic insufficiency, autoimmune factors, and certain NRTIs, have also been implicated in the pathogenesis of left ventricular dysfunction.[2,37] Therapeutic recommendations include standard therapy modalities for heart failure.[2] With the introduction of ART, there has been a significant decline in the prevalence of dilated cardiomyopathy.[35]

SUMMARY

The introduction of ART has markedly improved the prognosis of patients infected with HIV, changing the spectrum of cardiac disease in this population. Conditions such as dilated cardiomyopathy and pericardial diseases have become less common and CAD has become more common. HIV itself, and specific classes of ART such as PIs and certain NRTIs, may contribute to the development of CAD. Reflecting this susceptibility to accelerated coronary atherosclerosis, patients infected with HIV presenting with ACS are younger than the general population. The diagnostic and therapeutic approach to the patient with HIV presenting to the emergency department with ACS is the same as in the general population. With appropriate management of these acute manifestations of CAD, the prognosis for the patient infected with HIV is quite good.

REFERENCES

1. Boccara F. Cardiovascular complications and atherosclerotic manifestations in the HIV-infected population: type, incidence and associated risk factors. AIDS 2008;22(Suppl 3):S19–26.
2. Khunnawat C, Mukerji S, Havlichek D Jr, et al. Cardiovascular manifestations in human immunodeficiency virus-infected patients. Am J Cardiol 2008;102:635–42.
3. Holmberg SD, Moorman AC, Williamson JM, et al. Protease inhibitors and cardiovascular outcomes in patients with HIV-1. Lancet 2002;360:1747–8.
4. Klein D, Hurley LB, Quesenberry CP Jr, et al. Do protease inhibitors increase the risk for coronary heart disease in patients with HIV-1 infection? J Acquir Immune Defic Syndr 2002;30:471–7.
5. Bozzette SA, Ake CF, Tam HK, et al. Cardiovascular and cerebrovascular events in patients treated for human immunodeficiency virus infection. N Engl J Med 2003;348:702–10.
6. Mary-Krause M, Cotte L, Simon A, et al. Increased risk of myocardial infarction with duration of protease inhibitor therapy in HIV-infected men. AIDS 2003;17: 2479–86.
7. Friis-Moller N, Sabin CA, Weber R, et al. Combination antiretroviral therapy and the risk of myocardial infarction. N Engl J Med 2003;349:1993–2003.
8. d'Arminio A, Sabin CA, Phillips AN, et al. Cardio- and cerebrovascular events in HIV-infected persons. AIDS 2004;18:1811–7.
9. Friis-Moller N, Reiss P, Sabin CA, et al. Class of antiretroviral drugs and the risk of myocardial infarction. N Engl J Med 2007;356:1723–35.
10. The SMART/INSIGHT and the D:A:D Study Groups. Use of nucleoside reverse transcriptase inhibitors and risk of myocardial infarction in HIV-infected patients. AIDS 2008;22:F17–24.
11. Sabin CA, Worm SW, Weber R, et al. Use of nucleoside reverse transcriptase inhibitors and risk of myocardial infarction in HIV-infected patients enrolled in the D:A:D study: a multi-cohort collaboration. Lancet 2008;371:1417–26.
12. El-Sadr WM, Lundgren JD, Neaton JD, et al. CD4+ count-guided interruption of antiretroviral treatment. N Engl J Med 2006;355:2283–96.
13. Riddler SA, Smit E, Cole SR, et al. Impact of HIV infection and HAART on serum lipids in men. JAMA 2003;289:2978–82.
14. Mulligan K, Grunfeld C, Tai VW, et al. Hyperlipidemia and insulin resistance are induced by protease inhibitors independent of changes in body composition in patients with HIV infection. J Acquir Immune Defic Syndr 2000;23:35–43.

15. Grinspoon S, Carr A. Cardiovascular risk and body-fat abnormalities in HIV-infected adults. N Engl J Med 2005;352:48–62.
16. Martinez E, Mocroft A, Garcia-Viejo MA, et al. Risk of lipodystrophy in HIV-1-infected patients treated with protease inhibitors: a prospective cohort study. Lancet 2001;357:592–8.
17. Sattler FR, Qian D, Louie S, et al. Elevated blood pressure in subjects with lipodystrophy. AIDS 2001;15:2001–10.
18. Walli R, Herfort O, Michl GM, et al. Treatment with protease inhibitors associated with peripheral insulin resistance and impaired oral glucose tolerance in HIV-1-infected patients. AIDS 1998;12:F167–73.
19. Driscoll SD, Meininger GE, Lareau MT, et al. Effects of exercise training and metformin on body composition and cardiovascular indices in HIV-infected patients. AIDS 2004;18:465–73.
20. Fisher SD, Miller TL, Lipshultz SE. Impact of HIV and highly active antiretroviral therapy on leukocyte adhesion molecules, arterial inflammation, dyslipidemia, and atherosclerosis. Atherosclerosis 2006;185:1–11.
21. Ferry T, Raffi F, Collin-Filleul F, et al. Uncontrolled viral replication as a risk factor for non-AIDS severe clinical events in HIV-infected patients on long-term antiretroviral therapy: APROCO/COPILOTE (ANRS CO8) cohort study. J Acquir Immune Defic Syndr 2009;51:407–15.
22. Escaut L, Monsuez JJ, Chironi G, et al. Coronary artery disease in HIV infected patients. Intensive Care Med 2003;29:969–73.
23. Mehta NJ, Khan IA. HIV-associated coronary artery disease. Angiology 2003;54: 269–75.
24. Ambrose JA, Gould RB, Kurian DC, et al. Frequency of and outcome of acute coronary syndromes in patients with human immunodeficiency virus infection. Am J Cardiol 2003;92:301–3.
25. Hsue PY, Giri K, Erickson S, et al. Clinical features of acute coronary syndromes in patients with human immunodeficiency virus infection. Circulation 2004;109: 316–9.
26. Boccara F, Cohen A. Coronary artery disease and stroke in HIV-infected patients: prevention and pharmacological therapy. Adv Cardiol 2003;40:163–84.
27. Boccara F, Ederhy S, Janower S, et al. Clinical characteristics and mid-term prognosis of acute coronary syndrome in HIV-infected patients on antiretroviral therapy. HIV Med 2005;6:240–4.
28. Matetzky S, Domingo M, Kar S, et al. Acute myocardial infarction in human immunodeficiency virus-infected patients. Arch Intern Med 2003;163:457–60.
29. Boccara F, Teiger E, Cohen A, et al. Percutaneous coronary intervention in HIV infected patients: immediate results and long term prognosis. Heart 2006;92: 543–4.
30. Boccara F, Cohen A, Di Angelantonio E, et al. Coronary artery bypass graft in HIV-infected patients: a multicenter case control study. Curr HIV Res 2008;6: 59–64.
31. Heidenreich PA, Eisenberg MJ, Kee LL, et al. Pericardial effusion in AIDS. Incidence and survival. Circulation 1995;92:3229–34.
32. Hsia J, Ross AM. Pericardial effusion and pericardiocentesis in human immunodeficiency virus infection. Am J Cardiol 1994;74:94–6.
33. Silva-Cardoso J, Moura B, Martins L, et al. Pericardial involvement in human immunodeficiency virus infection. Chest 1999;115:418–22.
34. Barbaro G. Cardiovascular manifestations of HIV infection. Circulation 2002;106: 1420–5.

35. Pugliese A, Isnardi D, Saini A, et al. Impact of highly active antiretroviral therapy in HIV-positive patients with cardiac involvement. J Infect 2000;40:282–4.
36. Rerkpattanapipat P, Wongpraparut N, Jacobs LE, et al. Cardiac manifestations of acquired immunodeficiency syndrome. Arch Intern Med 2000;160:602–8.
37. Herskowitz A, Vlahov D, Willoughby S, et al. Prevalence and incidence of left ventricular dysfunction in patients with human immunodeficiency virus infection. Am J Cardiol 1993;71:955–8.
38. Currie PF, Jacob AJ, Foreman AR, et al. Heart muscle disease related to HIV infection: prognostic implications. BMJ 1994;309:1605–7.

Respiratory Emergencies in HIV-Infected Persons

Charles K. Everett, MD[a],*, Matthew W. Fei, MD[b],
Laurence Huang, MD[a],[c]

KEYWORDS

- HIV • Respiratory emergencies • Pneumonia
- PCP • Tuberculosis

Respiratory complaints are a common reason for patients with HIV infection to present to an emergency department (ED). "HIV and shortness of breath" is one of the most frequent chief complaints on ED triage sheets, and the differential diagnosis is broad. Pulmonary etiologies include infectious and noninfectious causes that are related and unrelated to underlying HIV infection and range from the minor (eg, upper respiratory infection [URI] and acute bronchitis) to the life threatening (eg, bacterial pneumonia and *Pneumocystis jiroveci* pneumonia [PCP]). This article focuses on respiratory emergencies among HIV-infected patients and discusses their typical presentation and diagnostic evaluation as well as therapeutic interventions that should be initiated in an ED.

EPIDEMIOLOGY

The cause of HIV-associated pulmonary disease partly depends on the setting in which patients are evaluated. The Pulmonary Complications of HIV Infection Study (PCHIS) was a prospective, observational cohort study that followed 1150 HIV-infected persons for 5 years at 6 centers in the United States. PCHIS found that HIV-infected individuals presenting to an outpatient setting with respiratory complaints more commonly had URIs and acute bronchitis, than lower respiratory tract infections, such as bacterial pneumonia and PCP.[1] In contrast, HIV-infected patients seeking care for their respiratory complaints in an ED are

[a] Division of Pulmonary and Critical Care Medicine, San Francisco General Hospital, University of California, San Francisco, 505 Parnassus Avenue, Box 0111, Room M1336, San Francisco, CA 94143, USA
[b] Division of Pulmonary and Critical Care Medicine, Bellevue Medical Center, 11511 NE 10th Street, Bellevue, WA 98004, USA
[c] Division of HIV/AIDS, San Francisco General Hospital, University of California, San Francisco, Ward 84, 995 Potrero Avenue, San Francisco, CA 94110, USA
* Corresponding author.
E-mail address: charles.everett@ucsf.edu

Emerg Med Clin N Am 28 (2010) 283–298
doi:10.1016/j.emc.2010.01.014
0733-8627/10/$ – see front matter © 2010 Elsevier Inc. All rights reserved.

more likely to present with serious illness, such as pneumonia, which often requires admission. In the authors' experience, patients who initiate contact with the health care system in an ED are less likely to have regular primary care for their HIV infection or to be on antiretroviral therapy (ART) or opportunistic infection (OI) prophylaxis, placing them at higher risk for life-threatening pulmonary disease.

The prevalence of pulmonary infections in HIV-infected persons is increased compared to the general population. In the absence of ART, the rate of bacterial pneumonia is between 5- and 25-fold higher in HIV-infected individuals than in the non-HIV infected population.[2,3] Although its prevalence has declined after the introduction of ART, PCP is still a common AIDS-defining illness and is seen almost exclusively in immunocompromised persons. Globally, Mycobacterium tuberculosis pneumonia (TB) is the major pulmonary infection complicating the HIV epidemic. In addition to HIV-associated opportunistic pneumonias, persons with HIV infection are at risk for HIV-associated neoplasms—Kaposi sarcoma and non-Hodgkin lymphoma—that may present with pulmonary involvement. Finally, emerging data indicate that HIV-infected persons are at an increased risk for noninfectious pulmonary conditions, including chronic obstructive pulmonary disease (COPD), lung cancer, and pulmonary arterial hypertension. A study conducted in France found that 33 of 147 patients with HIV presenting with acute respiratory failure requiring ICU admission had noninfectious causes for respiratory failure, and that proportion did not change over the 10 years studied.[4] Most notable among the noninfectious pulmonary conditions were pulmonary hypertension, pulmonary embolism, COPD exacerbation, and malignancy (AIDS- and non–AIDS-defining types). Patients with HIV are 50% to 60% more likely to have COPD than those without HIV.[5] They are 2.5 to 7.5 times more likely to have lung cancer, an effect seemingly related to the degree of immunosuppression.[6,7]

CLINICAL FEATURES

The clinical presentations of HIV-associated pulmonary diseases vary and often overlap. There is no pathognomonic finding that rules in or rules out a particular disease. The goal of a thorough history and physical is to narrow the differential diagnosis, recognize constellations of particular symptoms and signs, and guide diagnostic testing and therapy.

All of the HIV-associated pulmonary diseases can present with cough, shortness of breath, and decreased exercise tolerance. Fever is also common and typically points toward an infectious origin but can also be seen in noninfectious respiratory disease. Certain symptoms may lead a clinician to favor a particular diagnosis (Table 1). Purulent sputum is typically associated with bacterial pneumonia, whereas a dry, nonproductive cough is typically associated with PCP.[8] The duration of symptoms can also be useful in differentiating between pneumonias. Bacterial pneumonia characteristically presents with an acute onset over 3 to 5 days, whereas PCP and TB present with a more indolent onset over weeks to occasionally months. Although pleuritic chest pain can be observed in patients with any pulmonary infection, complaints of persistent, severe pleuritic pain should raise suspicion of a pneumothorax, particularly in patients with cysts and pneumatoceles secondary to PCP. Hemoptysis in the setting of fevers is frequently associated with tuberculosis, in particular if there is an indolent progression of disease, but more common causes are acute bacterial bronchitis and bacterial pneumonia. Hemoptysis should also raise the prospect of malignancy, in particular bronchogenic carcinoma, and pulmonary embolism.

The presence of extrapulmonary symptoms must also be noted, as these can be related to a primary pulmonary process and suggest a unifying diagnosis. A chronic history of constitutional symptoms, such as night sweats and weight loss, is common with TB infection but also is common with lymphoma. Lymphadenopathy, abdominal complaints, and organomegaly suggest infiltrative, granulomatous infection, such as TB, nontuberculous mycobacteria, and endemic fungal disease, or lymphoma. New-onset confusion, headache, or focal neurologic findings may indicate neurologic and pulmonary involvement by *Cryptococcus neoformans* or *Toxoplasma gondii*. Visual complaints and odynophagia may herald concurrent cytomegalovirus (CMV) retinitis, esophagitis, and pneumonitis. In these settings, biopsy of a peripheral lymph node, lumbar puncture, or dilated fundoscopic examination may yield the correct diagnosis.

More than 1 infectious agent may present concurrently in HIV-infected patients. Some patients have characteristics of dual respiratory infection with symptoms suggestive of a bacterial process and PCP or TB. For example, a patient who develops a cough productive of purulent sputum over several days may also complain of several weeks of fevers and dyspnea. Such a patient may have bacterial pneumonia superimposed on PCP. In these cases of suspected dual infection, empiric treatment of both processes is appropriate until a cause is determined. In one study, 22% of patients with HIV admitted to an ICU with respiratory failure had more than 1 cause; these patients had an increased risk for hospital mortality.[4]

Finally, consider noninfectious causes of an HIV-infected patient's respiratory complaints. The hallmarks of a COPD exacerbation in someone with HIV are no different from those in the general population: increased shortness of breath, wheeze, or cough; increase in the quantity of sputum production; or change in the quality of the sputum produced. Sudden onset of dyspnea and pleuritic chest pain may indicate pulmonary embolism. A prolonged history of dry cough with concomitant prominent weight loss suggests bronchogenic cancer. As discussed previously, hemoptysis may also be a clue. Kaposi sarcoma occasionally presents with isolated pulmonary involvement; the most common symptoms are cough, dyspnea, and fever.[9] All these diseases are more common in people with HIV.

PHYSICAL EXAMINATION

A thorough physical examination with emphasis on cardiopulmonary findings helps ED physicians narrow the differential diagnosis for HIV-infected patients with respiratory symptoms. Patients with HIV-associated pulmonary infections are typically febrile, tachycardic, and tachypneic. A decrease in oxygen saturation is frequent and is a common and appropriate indication for admission. If outpatient follow-up is considered, postambulation pulse oximetry should be checked, because some patients manifest hypoxia only after exertion.

The pulmonary examination should focus on the presence and characterization of focal or diffuse findings. Patients with bacterial pneumonia often have a focal lung examination suggestive of lobar consolidation with or without an accompanying pleural effusion. In contrast, patients with PCP may have diffuse but nonspecific findings with bilateral rales. It is common for patients with PCP to have a normal lung examination. The presence of diffuse wheezes can suggest an exacerbation of asthma, whereas decreased breath sounds may indicate COPD. The unilateral absence of breath sounds may suggest a pneumothorax in a patient complaining of pleuritic chest pain.

The remainder of the physical examination can be helpful in assessing patients' underlying immune status and the cause of their respiratory symptoms. PCP, bacterial pneumonia, and TB are often the HIV-identifying illnesses in patients who are unaware

Table 1
Presentation of common respiratory problems in HIV-infected patients

Clinical Features	
Bacterial Pneumonia	
Organisms	• *S pneumoniae* • *Haemophilus* species • Gram negative organisms and anaerobes (predisposing factors: alcohol use, aspiration)
Signs and symptoms	• Cough with purulent sputum • Fever, chills, rigors • Acute onset, symptoms <1 wk
Laboratory/radiographic tests	• Any CD4+ cell count • Elevated white blood cell count • Chest radiograph: unilateral focal alveolar consolidation, with or without associated pleural effusion
Clinical pearls	• Avoid fluoroquinolone therapy if high suspicion of *M tuberculosis*
PCP	
Signs and symptoms	• Nonproductive cough • Dyspnea • Fever • Gradual onset, symptoms >2 wk
Laboratory/radiographic tests	• CD4+ cell count: <200 cells/μL • Elevated serum LDH • Chest radiograph: bilateral reticular (interstitial) or granular pattern • HRCT: GGOs
Clinical pearls	• PCP can present with any pattern on chest radiograph, including a normal radiograph. If high clinical suspicion, consider empiric treatment while pursuing sputum induction, bronchoscopy, or HRCT
M tuberculosis	
Signs and symptoms	• Cough • Fever, night sweats • Weight loss • Gradual onset, symptoms >2 wk • Lymphadenopathy
Laboratory/radiographic tests	• Any CD4+ cell count • Chest radiograph: alveolar pattern (often with cavitation), miliary pattern, nodules, intrathoracic adenopathy, pleural effusion
Clinical pearls	• The characteristic pattern seen depends in part on the CD4+ cell count • Upper lung zone cavitary disease more common at higher CD4+ cell count • Alveolar infiltrate (mimicking bacterial pneumonia) or miliary pattern more common at lower CD4+ cell count

(continued on next page)

Table 1 (continued)	
Clinical Features	
Pulmonary Kaposi Sarcoma	
Signs and symptoms	• Cough • Dyspnea • Fever • Gradual onset, symptoms >2–4 wk
Laboratory/radiographic tests	• CD4+ cell count: <200 cells/μL • Chest radiograph: bilateral perihilar opacities, nodules, pleural effusion, intrathoracic adenopathy
Clinical pearls	• In the United States, most persons with pulmonary Kaposi sarcoma are men who have sex with men • Pulmonary Kaposi sarcoma can occasionally (15%) present in the absence of mucocutaneous involvement

of their underlying HIV infection. In addition to eliciting a history of potential HIV risk factors (men who have sex with men, injection drug use [IDU], or heterosexual sex for drugs or with sex workers), a physical examination may reveal oropharyngeal thrush. Lymphadenopathy may suggest disseminated mycobacterial or fungal disease or lymphoma. Skin and oropharyngeal examinations may reveal lesions consistent with Kaposi sarcoma or fungal disease.

LABORATORY AND RADIOGRAPHIC FINDINGS

The CD4+ cell count is essential in formulating a differential diagnosis in HIV-infected patients with respiratory symptoms. In cases where a patient is unaware of a recent CD4+ cell count, the total lymphocyte count can be obtained rapidly and serve as a surrogate marker, helping to estimate the degree of immune suppression. Acute illness can suppress the CD4+ cell count below the true baseline value, and a repeat CD4+ cell count after resolution of the acute illness may be indicated.

A room air arterial blood gas should be drawn in any patient with mild to moderate respiratory compromise or suspected PCP. A Pao_2 less than 70 mm Hg or an alveolar-arterial oxygen gradient greater than 35 mm Hg is an indication for adjunctive corticosteroid treatment in PCP. Serum lactate dehydrogenase (LDH) is another laboratory test that has prognostic importance in PCP. LDH is frequently, but not invariably, elevated in patients infected with PCP, and the degree of elevation correlates with prognosis.[8] A baseline LDH value can help assess severity of illness and also assist an admitting physician should a patient's clinical status worsen. In addition to these and other more common laboratory tests (eg, complete blood count and metabolic panels), an electrocardiogram should be obtained to evaluate for cardiac disease as the potential cause of respiratory symptoms (**Table 2**).

The authors recommend that all HIV-infected patients who present with a suspected pulmonary infection have 2 sets of blood cultures drawn in an ED prior to initiating antibiotic therapy. Although current joint guidelines for community-acquired pneumonia from the Infectious Diseases Society of America and the American Thoracic Society do not categorically recommend blood cultures for all patients with HIV and suspected pneumonia, the vast majority presenting to an ED meet the criteria for blood cultures set out in those guidelines.[10] Similar to non–HIV-infected patients, in HIV-infected patients, *Streptococcus pneumoniae* is the most common cause of bacterial

Table 2 Standard ED evaluation for HIV-infected patients with suspected pulmonary infection	
All patients	• CD4+ cell count (if unknown or last value >6 mo ago) • Complete blood count with differential and metabolic panel • Chest radiograph (posteroanterior and lateral)—compare with prior radiograph • Electrocardiogram
Selected patients	• Room air arterial blood gas (if patient has mild to moderate respiratory compromise or if PCP is suspected) • Serum LDH (if PCP is suspected) • Sputum Gram stain and culture (if bacterial pneumonia is suspected) • Blood cultures (2 sets prior to antibiotic administration if bacterial pneumonia is suspected) • Serum cryptococcal antigen (if CD4+ cell count <200 cells/μL)

pneumonia, and in patients with lower CD4+ cell counts, bacteremia is more frequent. Positive blood cultures with subsequent antibiotic susceptibility testing help guide appropriate antimicrobial therapy. In addition, HIV-infected patients may have more than 1 bacterial process at the same time given their immune suppression and other risk factors (eg, IDU).

If a bacterial respiratory infection is suspected and a patient has a productive cough, a sputum sample should be sent for Gram stain and culture. Prior antibiotic administration can decrease the sensitivity of sputum bacterial culture, but a Gram stain may still yield useful information, especially if the sample is sent expeditiously to a laboratory for analysis. Although the sensitivity of a sputum culture for bacterial pneumonia is widely variable (approximately 40%–80%), isolating a pathogen from sputum with subsequent antibiotic susceptibility testing can help guide therapy.[10]

In addition to bacterial Gram stain and culture, sputum should be sent for PCP stain and acid fast bacilli (AFB) in the proper clinical scenarios. Most patients with PCP alone (without a superimposed bacterial pneumonia) have a nonproductive cough and are unable to produce a spontaneously expectorated sputum sample. In these cases, sputum induction using nebulized hypertonic saline should be performed. The sensitivity of sputum induction varies depending on the method used, the institution, and the prevalence of PCP but can reach 74% to 92% in experienced centers.[11,12] In patients suspected of having TB, expectorated or induced sputum for AFB should be collected daily for 3 consecutive days while patients are in respiratory isolation. The sensitivity of sputum AFB smears for M tuberculosis ranges from 50% to 60% and can approach 90% in those with disseminated disease.[13,14] Three negative AFB smears do not rule out active TB, but the likelihood of airborne transmission to other patients and health care providers is significantly decreased. Therefore, these patients can be removed from respiratory isolation while awaiting the results of AFB culture.

There are caveats to sputum collection for PCP and AFB. Patients who are recently diagnosed with PCP and have undergone a complete course of treatment may continue to have positive sputum stains for PCP despite resolution of infection.[15] This can make a diagnosis of recurrent respiratory complaints problematic, because these patients may have inadequately treated PCP or a second infectious pulmonary process. A positive sputum AFB smear is not synonymous with M tuberculosis and can be due to colonization or infection by nontuberculous mycobacteria, such as M avium complex. Nevertheless, any positive AFB smear must be approached as if it represents M tuberculosis, and appropriate infection control and treatment measures must be implemented until a definitive diagnosis is made. In the authors' experience, it may be impractical to have sputum induction routinely performed in an ED because of time constraints and the lack of properly engineered rooms.

CHEST RADIOGRAPH

Although there are characteristic chest radiograph findings for common HIV-associated pulmonary infections, overlap does occur between different disease processes. A basic interpretation of chest radiographs can be accomplished in an ED by assessing the following: (1) normal or abnormal—if abnormal, (2) pattern of disease (eg, alveolar, interstitial, or nodular), (3) distribution of disease (eg, unilateral or bilateral, focal, or diffuse), and (4) associated findings (eg, pleural effusion, mediastinal or hilar adenopathy, pneumatocele, or cavitation). Because HIV-infected patients may present with several different respiratory infections over time, leading to residual chest radiographic findings, it is critical to compare the current radiograph against prior radiographs, especially the most recent ones.

Bacterial pneumonia is the most common pulmonary infection in HIV-infected patients in the United States. Characteristic findings are similar to those in the non–HIV-infected population, with unilateral focal, lobar, or segmental alveolar infiltrates predominating (**Fig. 1**). In contrast, *Haemophilus influenzae* pneumonia seems to have a higher likelihood of presenting with an interstitial pattern that mimics PCP.[16]

A characteristic radiograph in PCP has bilateral, diffuse interstitial, reticular, or granular opacities (**Fig. 2**). The findings can be unilateral or asymmetric. Patients with PCP can present with pneumatoceles in 10% to 20% of cases or can develop them as treatment progresses. Pneumatoceles vary in number and size and place patients at increased risk for pneumothorax. A normal chest radiograph or one with focal lobar consolidation does not rule out PCP.[17] PCP should be high on the differential diagnosis in a HIV-infected patient with a CD4+ cell count less than 200 cells/μL who is hypoxemic, febrile, and has a normal chest radiograph. In addition, an apical pattern mimicking TB can be seen, classically in patients on aerosolized pentamidine

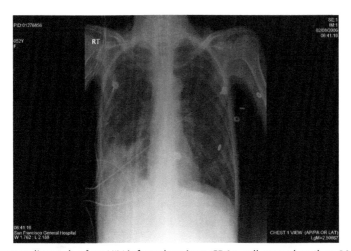

Fig. 1. Chest radiograph of an HIV-infected patient, CD4+ cell count less than 200 cells/μL, with lobar consolidation from *S pneumoniae*. This patient was also found to have *S pneumoniae* bacteremia, meningitis, and *Staphylococcus aureus* bacteremia. (*Courtesy of Laurence Huang, MD.*)

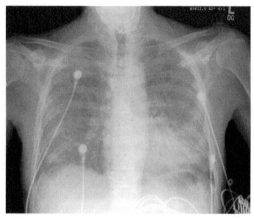

Fig. 2. Chest radiograph of an HIV-infected patient, CD4+ cell count less than 200 cells/μL, demonstrating the bilateral, reticular pattern characteristic of PCP. Bronchoscopy with bronchoalveolar lavage fluid examination revealed PCP. (*Courtesy of* Laurence Huang, MD.)

prophylaxis. Intrathoracic adenopathy and pleural effusions are rare in PCP, however, and these findings should prompt a search for and treatment of an alternate (or coexisting) process.

Like PCP, *M tuberculosis* can present with a variety of radiographic findings, including a normal chest radiograph. The specific pattern seen often correlates with a patient's degree of immune suppression, so knowledge of the most recent CD4+ cell count is helpful. TB developing early in the course of HIV infection (ie, high CD4+ count) typically presents with a pattern of classic reactivation disease, with cavitating infiltrates in the upper lung zones (**Fig. 3**). TB developing in the later stages of HIV infection (ie, low CD4+ count) often presents with middle and lower lung zone infiltrates and less frequently presents with cavitation (**Fig. 4**). This radiographic picture can imitate a bacterial pneumonia.

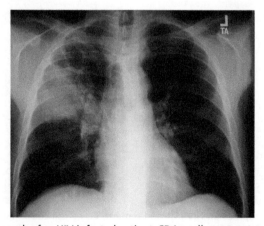

Fig. 3. Chest radiograph of an HIV-infected patient, CD4+ cell count greater than 200 cells/μL, revealing right upper lobe infiltrate with areas of cavitation. Sputum AFB stain was positive and multiple sputum AFB cultures grew *M tuberculosis*. (*Courtesy of* Laurence Huang, MD.)

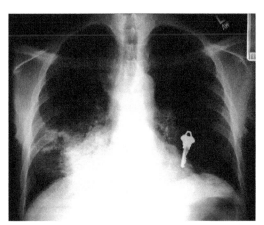

Fig. 4. Chest radiograph of an HIV-infected patient, CD4+ cell count less than 200 cells/μL, revealing right lower lung consolidation with air bronchograms. Sputum AFB cultures grew *M tuberculosis* that was monorifampin resistant. In this case, the key to the diagnosis of TB was knowledge of the patient's CD4+ cell count and an understanding that TB can present in this manner in such an individual. (*Courtesy of* Laurence Huang, MD.)

CHEST CT

Chest CT can be useful in the diagnosis of suspected PCP when a plain radiograph is normal or unchanged. In this setting, a high-resolution CT (HRCT) serves as a sensitive diagnostic study for PCP. Patients with PCP and a normal chest radiograph have patchy areas of ground-glass opacities (GGOs) on HRCT (**Fig. 5**). Although the presence of GGOs is nonspecific, their absence strongly argues against a diagnosis of PCP.[18] In addition, CT is helpful for evaluation of associated findings, such as pleural

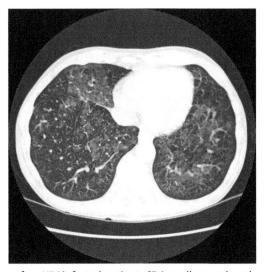

Fig. 5. Chest CT scan of an HIV-infected patient, CD4+ cell count less than 200 cells/μL, with GGOs characteristic of PCP. Induced sputum examination revealed PCP. (*Courtesy of* Laurence Huang, MD.)

effusion, intrathoracic adenopathy, pulmonary nodules, and cavitation, and helps guide further diagnostic and therapeutic procedures directed at findings, including chest tube placement or lymph node biopsy.

DIFFERENTIAL DIAGNOSIS

When evaluating HIV-infected patients with respiratory symptoms, consider infectious and noninfectious causes of cough, dyspnea, and hypoxia. Given an appropriate past medical history, exacerbations of underlying asthma or COPD are common. HIV can be a cause of cardiac dysfunction, and HIV-associated cardiomyopathy and pulmonary arterial hypertension are important diagnoses to consider in patients with compatible findings on examination (eg, elevated jugular venous pressure and rales) and chest radiography (eg, cardiomegaly and pulmonary edema). Apart from AIDS-defining malignancies, such as Kaposi sarcoma and non-Hodgkin lymphoma, both of which can present with respiratory symptoms, be alert to complications of primary lung cancer, such as pleural effusion, airway obstruction, and postobstructive pneumonia.

The distinction between infectious and noninfectious causes of pulmonary disease in HIV-infected patients usually becomes evident after a thorough history, physical examination, and basic diagnostic tests. Patients with common and uncommon pulmonary infections typically complain of fever, cough (with or without purulent sputum), dyspnea, night sweats, fatigue, decreased exercise tolerance, and weight loss of varying duration. The most common causes of pulmonary infection necessitating an ED visit and subsequent admission in HIV-infected patients are bacterial pneumonia followed by PCP, both of which are significantly more common than the next most common diagnoses: TB, pulmonary Kaposi sarcoma (associated with human herpesvirus 8), and various fungal infections.

Patient social and travel history also factors into the likelihood of a particular infection causing respiratory disease. The probability of presenting with pneumonia due to an endemic fungus can be ascertained with a careful travel history. Other respiratory diseases can be associated with mode of HIV transmission. In the United States, Kaposi sarcoma is almost exclusively seen in men who have sex with men.[9] Primary or reactivation of *M tuberculosis* infection is associated with homelessness, incarceration, recent immigration from an endemic country, and recent conversion to a positive tuberculin skin test, defined as greater than or equal to 5-mm induration in HIV-infected persons.[19] Those with IDU have a higher rate of bacterial pneumonia and TB than persons who have no history of IDU.[2]

CD4+ Cell Count

An essential component in formulating a differential diagnosis is patients' most recent CD4+ cell count and their history of prior OIs. Equally important to narrowing the differential diagnosis is patients' use of and adherence to ART and OI prophylaxis. The CD4+ cell count is still an excellent indicator of an HIV-infected patients' susceptibility to opportunistic respiratory infections (**Table 3**).

Some pulmonary infections, such as bacterial pneumonia and TB, can occur at any CD4+ count, but both are more frequent and have an increasing complication rate as the CD4+ cell count declines. At lower CD4+ cell counts, bacteremia accompanying bacterial pneumonia becomes increasingly common and TB is often disseminated. Other opportunistic respiratory infections occur predominantly at a CD4+ cell count less than 200 cells/μL. At this level, PCP and cryptococcal pneumonia enter the differential diagnosis, whereas neither is commonly seen at counts than 200 cells/μL. At

Table 3	
Differential diagnosis of respiratory infections in HIV/AIDS	
Any CD4+ cell count	• Bacterial pneumonia (most commonly *S pneumoniae* or *H influenzae*) • TB
CD4+ <200 cells/μL	• PCP • *Cryptococcus neoformans* pneumonia • Bacterial pneumonia complicated by bacteremia • Extrapulmonary or disseminated TB
CD4+ <100 cells/μL	• *P aeruginosa* pneumonia • *Toxoplasma gondii* pneumonia • Pulmonary Kaposi sarcoma
CD4+ <50 cells/μL	• *Histoplasma capsulatum* or *C immitis* pneumonia, usually associated with disseminated disease • CMV pneumonia, usually associated with disseminated disease • *M avium* complex pneumonia, usually associated with disseminated disease • *Aspergillus* species pneumonia

a CD4+ cell count less than 100 cells/μL, pulmonary Kaposi sarcoma, *Toxoplasma gondii*, and *Pseudomonas aeruginosa* pneumonias can be seen. As the CD4+ cell count drops below 50 cells/μL, the endemic fungi (*Histoplasma capsulatum* and *Coccidioides immitis*), *Aspergillus* species, CMV, and nontuberculous mycobacteria become considerations for pulmonary infection. The CD4+ cell count should serve as a general guideline as exceptions can occur (see **Table 3**).

Unfortunately, patients presenting to an ED may not have had a recent CD4+ cell count. In these cases, an ED physician needs to look for surrogate markers of suppressed immune function. Finding oropharyngeal thrush (candidiasis) on physical examination may be an indication of underlying immunocompromise. A history of thrush also increases the risk of subsequent PCP.

Prior Respiratory Illness and Use of OI Prophylaxis

Many of the HIV-associated OIs have a tendency to recur. Recurrent bacterial pneumonia (eg, 2 or more episodes in a 12-month period) was added to the list of AIDS-defining illnesses in the 1993 Centers for Disease Control and Prevention expanded surveillance case definition for AIDS.[20] Patients with a history of PCP and fungal infections (cryptococcosis, coccidioidomycosis, and histoplasmosis) are also at high risk for recurrent illness, especially if they fail to take secondary prophylaxis/maintenance therapy.[21] Although respiratory symptoms in an HIV-infected patient can be due to a new infectious process, clinicians should be aware of patients' prior history given the high likelihood of relapsed infection.

HIV-infected patients, especially those with the lowest CD4+ cell counts, may develop an OI despite the use of antimicrobial prophylaxis. When evaluating a patient with HIV infection, CD4+ cell counts and adherence to OI prophylaxis should serve as a general guide as to which pulmonary infections are most likely to occur in a patient. Exceptions to the rule can and do occur.

ADMISSION CRITERIA

In addition to triage, the role of ED physicians in the care of HIV-infected patients with a respiratory emergency is to initiate an appropriate diagnostic work-up such that a definitive diagnosis can be made expeditiously. As discussed previously, many of the HIV-associated pulmonary diseases can resemble each other by history, physical examination, laboratory testing, and radiographic imaging. HIV-associated pulmonary infections, in particular, have the potential to progress rapidly to respiratory failure and death in the absence of appropriate therapy. In addition, therapies for many of the OIs have significant toxicities and may have important drug-drug interactions with other HIV medications, including ART. Additional considerations include the stability of a patient's social situation and ability to seek follow-up medical care (**Table 4**).

Thus, patients who have an established primary care physician, a CD4+ cell count greater than 200 cells/μL, and normal pulse oximetry after ambulation and who are suspected of having bacterial pneumonia by history and radiographic imaging could potentially be discharged home on appropriate empiric antibiotic therapy with close follow-up. Patients, however, with a CD4+ cell count less than 200 cells/μL or a history or imaging studies suspicious for PCP or TB should be admitted for diagnostic work-up, unless diagnostic testing (sputum induction and potentially bronchoalveolar lavage) can be arranged as outpatients in an expedited manner. Discharging patients on empiric therapy for a presumed diagnosis of PCP without any plans to establish a definitive microbiologic diagnosis can be problematic and is seldom justified.

TREATMENT

It is recommended that medical providers begin empiric antibiotics for suspected pulmonary infection before a definitive diagnosis has been made.

Regarding infectious causes, what is appropriate initial treatment of a nonspecific illness? The answer depends on the pretest probability of disease, which is based on patient CD4+ cell count, history, physical examination, and imaging studies. As the most common causes of HIV-associated pulmonary infection are bacterial pneumonia and PCP, empiric therapy for 1 or both pneumonias is often implemented. A typical patient with bacterial pneumonia may present with the following: CD4+

Table 4	
High risk for clinical deterioration in HIV-infected patients with suspected pulmonary infection	
High risk for clinical deterioration	• Tachypnea with respiratory rate >25 breaths per min • Hypotension with systolic blood pressure persistently <90 mm Hg after initial fluid resuscitation • Hypoxia with decreased Pao_2, elevated alveolar-arterial oxygen gradient, or requiring supplemental oxygen; oxygen desaturation with exertion • CD4+ cell count <200 cells/μL • Decreased exercise tolerance with limited ability to perform independent daily activities • General ill appearance • Coexisting medical or psychiatric disease that potentially increases severity of pulmonary infection or decreases likelihood of outpatient treatment adherence • Marginal social situation (ie, homeless or substance abuse)
Potential for infection transmission	• Suspected active tuberculosis and with risk of transmission to other individuals at place of residence
Other	• Inability to provide appropriate follow up (eg, no primary care provider) • Inability to schedule necessary diagnostic testing (eg, sputum induction or bronchoscopy)

cell count greater than 200 cells/μL; chest radiograph with a noncavitating focal, segmental, or lobar infiltrate; and a history of 3 to 5 days of fevers, rigors, and cough productive of purulent sputum. Other suggestive factors include focal findings on lung examination, leukocytosis, and a history of cigarette smoking, IDU, or prior bacterial pneumonia. Given the constellation of findings in these patients, the pretest probability of bacterial pneumonia is significantly higher than of PCP or TB. Empiric therapy for bacterial pneumonia alone is appropriate pending further diagnostic testing (Tables 5 and 6). The US Public Health Service guidelines for treatment and prevention of OIs make recommendations for HIV-infected patients with bacterial pneumonia. In general, a hospitalized patient with mild to moderate respiratory compromise should be treated with an extended-spectrum cephalosporin (ceftriaxone or cefotaxime) and a macrolide or doxycycline or an antipneumococcal fluoroquinolone (eg, levofloxacin). For patients with severe respiratory compromise or patients requiring ICU admission, combination therapy with an extended-spectrum cephalosporin and azithromycin or a fluoroquinolone should be instituted, with a goal of providing optimal therapy for the 2 most commonly identified causes of lethal pneumonia (S pneumoniae and Legionella species).[10] In cases where the clinical scenario suggests a bacterial pneumonia but could potentially be TB, the authors recommend avoiding the use of fluoroquinolones until TB has been ruled in or out. Multidrug-resistant TB in HIV-infected patients remains a serious concern and fluoroquinolones are a mainstay of TB therapy

Table 5	
Management of respiratory infection in patients with HIV/AIDS and CD4+ cell count (known or suspected) <200 cells/μL	
Acute Symptoms (<1 Wk)	
Normal chest radiograph	• Symptomatic treatment of URI • Arrange follow-up with primary provider • If symptoms persist or progress, consider repeat chest radiograph or HRCT to evaluate for PCP
Abnormal chest radiograph	• Bacterial pneumonia > PCP, TB • Consider admission for antibiotics and further evaluation for PCP or TB if risk factors present (eg, prior PCP or homeless) or mixed clinical picture (eg, nonproductive cough or severe dyspnea) that are more suggestive of PCP
Chronic Symptoms (>1 Wk)	
Normal chest radiograph or interstitial infiltrate	Nonproductive cough • PCP > bacterial pneumonia, TB • Evaluate for PCP (and possibly TB) with induced sputum, bronchoscopy • Empiric treatment of PCP while awaiting diagnostic testing Productive cough • Mixed clinical picture: consider empiric treatment of both bacterial pneumonia and PCP while awaiting further diagnostic testing
Alveolar infiltrate	Nonproductive cough • Mixed clinical picture: consider empiric treatment of both bacterial pneumonia and PCP while awaiting further diagnostic testing Productive cough • Bacterial pneumonia > PCP or TB • Consider treatment with antibiotics of bacterial pneumonia and further evaluation for PCP and TB

Table 6
Treatment of common HIV-related pulmonary infections

Infection	Preferred Therapy	Alternative Therapies/Other Issues
PCP[19]	1. TMP/SMX: 15–20 mg TMP/kg body weight daily IV divided q6–8h; or 2. Same daily dose of TMP/SMX (based on TMP) po divided q8h; or 3. TMP/SMX ds 2 tablets po q8h Total duration 21 d AND Prednisone 40 mg bid d 1–5, 40 mg daily d 6–10, then 20 mg daily d 11–21, if Pao$_2$ <70 mm Hg at room air or alveolar-arterial O$_2$ gradient >35 mm Hg	1. Primaquine 15–30 mg (base) po daily and clindamycin 600–900 mg IV q6–8h or Clindamycin 300–450 mg po q6–8h; or 2. Dapsone 100 mg po daily and TMP 5 mg/kg po q8h; or 3. Atovaquone 750 mg po bid; or 4. Pentamidine 3–4 mg/kg IV daily
M tuberculosis[19,20]	Isoniazid 5 mg/kg (max: 300 mg) po daily and rifampin 10 mg/kg (max: 600 mg) po daily and PZA and EMB; PZA and EMB dose based on weight[a]	Urgent initiation of TB therapy in an ED is rarely necessary Consultation with infectious disease specialist or pharmacist recommended due to multiple drug interactions between TB therapy and ART
Bacterial pneumonia[5,6,19]	Empiric therapy targeting S pneumoniae and H influenzae 1. Mild to moderate disease: second- or third-generation cephalosporin and macrolide or doxycycline or antipneumococcal fluoroquinolone 2. Severe disease: second- or third-generation cephalosporin and macrolide or fluoroquinolone	Minimize use of fluoroquinolones unless there is no suspicion of TB; fluoroquinolones should be reserved for treatment of drug-resistant TB and in TB patients with liver disease

Abbreviations: EMB, ethambutol; IV, intravenous; max, maximum; PZA, pyrazinamide; SMX, sulfamethoxazole; TMP, trimethoprim.
  [a] PZA dose: <55 kg = 1000 mg; 56–75 kg = 1500 mg; >75 kg = 2000 mg; EMB dose: <55 kg = 800 mg; 56–75 kg = 1200 mg; >75 kg = 1600 mg.

in this clinical scenario. All efforts must be made to prevent the development of fluoroquinolone resistance in multidrug-resistant TB.[22]

A second case scenario involves an HIV-infected patient with a CD4+ cell count of less than 200 cells/μL. As the CD4+ cell count declines, the number of possible diagnoses increases, although bacterial pneumonia and PCP remain the 2 most common causes. If a chest radiograph shows a focal alveolar infiltrate and other findings are consistent with bacterial pneumonia, empiric treatment of common bacterial pathogens alone is reasonable. If a chest radiograph reveals bilateral reticular, interstitial, or granular opacities and a patient describes a subacute onset of fevers, dyspnea, and dry cough accompanied by an elevated serum LDH, PCP is the most likely diagnosis. Empiric therapy with trimethoprim/sulfamethoxazole and corticosteroids (if indicated by a Pao$_2$ <70 mm Hg on room air or alveolar-arterial oxygen gradient >35 mm Hg) should be instituted while arranging for sputum induction or bronchoscopy to diagnose PCP. In reality, clinical medicine rarely follows classic textbook descriptions, and it is common for patients to present with features consistent with both bacterial pneumonia and PCP (eg, subacute onset of fevers but cough productive of purulent sputum). Therefore, it is reasonable and common to begin empiric therapy for both bacterial pneumonia and PCP while pursuing further testing to arrive at a definitive diagnosis.

ISOLATION AND INFECTION CONTROL

The transmission of infectious respiratory disease between HIV-infected patients and health care workers in hospitals is a significant concern. An active cough and certain medical procedures (eg, endotracheal intubation, sputum induction, and bronchoscopy) increase the burden of airborne bacilli and thus infectious risk. As described previously, the clinical and radiographic presentations of pulmonary TB in the setting of HIV infection are myriad. ED physicians must also assess HIV-infected patients with respiratory symptoms for the possibility of active pulmonary TB. All suspected cases of TB must be placed in respiratory isolation (preferably negative pressure respiratory isolation). Appropriate precautions, such as use of N95 face masks, should be implemented by hospital staff in contact with suspected cases of TB until 2 to 3 separate sputum specimens have been examined and are negative for AFB. Given the myriad radiographic and clinical presentations of tuberculosis in HIV-infected patients, ED physicians must have a low threshold for placing suspected patients in respiratory isolation.

SUMMARY

When evaluating patients with HIV and respiratory symptoms, the differential diagnosis is broad and includes infectious and noninfectious causes that can be related or unrelated to underlying HIV infection. Consider risk factors for noninfectious pulmonary disease, such as smoking, or known comorbidities, such as COPD, when assessing for a non-HIV related cause of respiratory distress. A patient's CD4+ cell count, history of prior OI, and adherence to ART and OI prophylaxis are essential in helping to narrow the differential diagnosis for HIV-associated pulmonary infections. M tuberculosis and bacterial pneumonia can occur with any CD4+ cell count. The 2 most common HIV-associated pulmonary infections are bacterial pneumonia and PCP. A thorough history, physical examination, and review of chest radiograph are often helpful in differentiating between these 2 infections. The classic chest radiograph for PCP is a diffuse, bilateral, reticular (interstitial), or granular infiltrates. PCP can also manifest, however, as a focal airspace opacity or a normal chest radiograph. When considering criteria for admission, ED physicians must remember that establishing a definitive diagnosis is preferable to empiric outpatient therapy for most HIV-associated pulmonary infections, given the likelihood for rapid respiratory decompensation in this patient population.

REFERENCES

1. Wallace JM, Hansen NI, Lavange L, et al. Respiratory disease trends in the Pulmonary Complications of HIV Infection Study cohort. Pulmonary Complications of HIV Infection Study Group. Am J Respir Crit Care Med 1997;155(1):72–80.
2. Hirschtick RE, Glassroth J, Jordan MC, et al. Bacterial pneumonia in persons infected with the human immunodeficiency virus. N Engl J Med 1995;333:845–51.
3. Feikin D, Feldman C, Schuchat A, et al. Global strategies to prevent bacterial pneumonia in adults with HIV disease. Lancet Infect Dis 2004;4:445–55.

4. Barbier F, Coquet I, Legriel S, et al. Etiologies and outcome of acute respiratory failure in HIV-infected patients. Intensive Care Med 2009;35(10):1678–86.
5. Crothers K, Butt AA, Gibert CL, et al. Increased COPD among HIV-positive compared to HIV-negative veterans. Chest 2006;130(5):1326–33.
6. Barbaro G, Barbarini G. HIV infection and cancer in the era of highly active anti-retroviral therapy. Oncol Rep 2007;17:1121–6.
7. Frisch M, Biggar RJ, Engels EA, et al. Association of cancer with AIDS-related immunosuppression in adults. JAMA 2001;285:1736–45.
8. Huang L, Stansell JD. AIDS and the lung. Med Clin North Am 1996;80(4):775–801.
9. Huang L, Schnapp LM, Gruden JF, et al. Presentation of AIDS-related pulmonary Kaposi's sarcoma diagnosed by bronchoscopy. Am J Respir Crit Care Med 1996; 153(4 Pt 1):1385–90.
10. Mandell LA, Wunderink RG, Ansueto A, et al. Infectious Disease Society of America/American Thoracic Society Consensus Guidelines on the management of community-acquired pneumonia in adults. Clin Infect Dis 2007;44:S27–72.
11. Turner D, Schwarz Y, Yust I. Induced sputum for diagnosing Pneumocystis carinii pneumonia in HIV patients: new data, new issues. Eur Respir J 2003;21:204–8.
12. Hadley WK, Ng VL. Organization of microbiology laboratory services for the diagnosis of pulmonary infections in patients with human immunodeficiency virus infection. Semin Respir Infect 1989;2:85–92.
13. Greenberg SD, Frager D, Suster B, et al. Active pulmonary tuberculosis in patients with AIDS: spectrum of radiographic findings (including a normal appearance). Radiology 1994;193(1):115–9.
14. Smith RL, Yew K, Berkowitz KA, et al. Factors affecting the yield of acid-fast sputum smears in patients with HIV and tuberculosis. Chest 1994;106(3):684–6.
15. O'Donnell WJ, Pieciak W, Chertow GM, et al. Clearance of Pneumocystis carinii cysts in acute P carinii pneumonia: assessment by serial sputum induction. Chest 1998;114(5):1264–8.
16. Moreno S, Martinez R, Barros C, et al. Latent Haemophilus influenzae pneumonia in patients infected with HIV. AIDS 1991;5(8):967–70.
17. Kennedy CA, Goetz MB. Atypical roentgenographic manifestations of Pneumocystis carinii pneumonia. Arch Intern Med 1992;152(7):1390–8.
18. Gruden JF, Huang L, Turner J, et al. High-resolution CT in the evaluation of clinically suspected Pneumocystis carinii pneumonia in AIDS patients with normal, equivocal, or nonspecific radiographic findings. AJR Am J Roentgenol 1997; 169(4):967–75.
19. Targeted tuberculin testing and treatment of latent tuberculosis infection. American Thoracic Society and the Centers for Disease Control and Prevention. Am J Respir Crit Care Med 2000;161(4 Pt 2):S221–47.
20. Centers for Disease Control and Prevention. From the Centers for Disease Control and Prevention. 1993 revised classification system for HIV infection and expanded surveillance case definition for AIDS among adolescents and adults. JAMA 1993;269(6):729–30.
21. Kaplan JE, Benson C, Holmes KH, et al. Centers for Disease Control and Prevention. Guidelines for the prevention and treatment of opportunistic infections in HIV-infected adults and adolescents. MMWR Recomm Rep 2009;58. (No. RR-4):1–207.
22. Wells CD, Cegielski JP, Nelson LJ, et al. HIV and multi-drug resistant tuberculosis—the perfect storm. J Infect Dis 2007;196:S86–107.

Diarrhea in Patients Infected with HIV Presenting to the Emergency Department

George W. Beatty, MD, MPH

KEYWORDS
- Diarrhea • Gastrointestinal manifestations
- Opportunistic infections

Diarrhea is an exceedingly common complaint in patients with human immunodeficiency virus (HIV) infection, and the severity of symptoms ranges from mild, self-limiting diarrhea to debilitating disease that can result in malnutrition, volume loss, and shock. Up to 40% of patients with HIV infection report at least one episode of diarrhea in a given month, and approximately one quarter of patients experience chronic diarrhea at some point.[1] The prevalence of diarrhea increases with decreasing CD4 counts. More than 50% of patients with a CD4 count less than 50 cells/mm^3 will experience at least one episode of diarrhea each year, and in some areas this number will approach 100%. Approximately one-half of patients hospitalized with complications of HIV infection report diarrhea. Diarrhea has been shown to be an independent predictor of death in this population.[2]

CLINICAL FEATURES AND DIAGNOSIS

A useful initial approach to evaluating diarrhea in an individual infected with HIV is to distinguish between acute and chronic diarrhea, and between small and large bowel involvement (**Table 1** and **Boxes 1** and **2**). Particular consideration should also be given to the stage of HIV disease, current medications, and sexual history, as these factors help determine likely pathogens. Evaluating the degree of systemic illness is essential to assessing the need for hospital admission.

Acute diarrhea is defined as the presence of 3 or more loose or watery stools per day for 3 days to 2 weeks. Diarrhea is defined as persistent if it has been present between 2 and 4 weeks, and is considered chronic when present for 4 weeks or

Department of Medicine, University of California San Francisco, Building 80, Ward 84, 995 Potrero Avenue, San Francisco, CA 94110, USA
E-mail address: gbeatty@php.ucsf.edu

Emerg Med Clin N Am 28 (2010) 299–310
doi:10.1016/j.emc.2010.01.003
0733-8627/10/$ – see front matter © 2010 Elsevier Inc. All rights reserved.

Table 1
Small versus large bowel diarrhea

	Symptoms	Common Pathogens
Small bowel	• Large volume • Watery stool • Upper abdominal cramps • Bloating • Gas • Weight loss • Malnutrition • Dehydration	• Salmonella[a] • E coli • Viral (eg, rotavirus) • Giardia • MAC • Cryptosporidium[a] • Microsporidium[a] • Malabsorption
Large bowel	• Small volumes • Frequent bowel movements • Mucoid or bloody stool • Tenesmus • Lower abdominal cramps	• Yersinia • Campylobacter[a] • Shigella • C difficile • CMV • Enteroinvasive E coli • Entamoeba histolytica • Gonorrhea

[a] May involve both small and large bowel, but typically presents as listed.

more. Pathogens infecting the small bowel affect the secretory and nutritional absorptive functions of the gastrointestinal tract, and typically present with large volumes of watery stool, often accompanied by cramps, bloating, and abdominal gas. If the diarrhea is severe or prolonged, dehydration, malnutrition, and weight loss may manifest. Large bowel involvement primarily affects water resorptive capacity and typically causes frequent, small-volume diarrhea that may be bloody or mucoid and is often accompanied by pain.

In general, diarrheal symptoms are nonspecific in patients infected with HIV, as they are in the host without HIV infection.[3] Patients with bacterial diarrhea often, although not invariably, present with associated crampy abdominal pain.[4] The lack of associated abdominal pain or other symptoms should suggest viral acute gastroenteritis (AGE) or medication side effects. In patients with the large-volume watery diarrhea characteristic of small bowel infections, volume loss may result in dizziness, syncope, pallor, electrolyte imbalances (hypokalemia, hyponatremia), and acute renal insufficiency. Signs of invasive or systemic involvement include the presence of fever, severe abdominal cramps, and bloody stools. Patients with long-standing chronic diarrhea may exhibit obvious wasting or malnutrition, but these may also result from advanced HIV infection.[5]

Diarrhea in patients infected with HIV poses a diagnostic dilemma in the acute care setting, as these patients are susceptible to all of the infections associated with diarrhea in the normal host, as well as a multitude of opportunistic infections and medication side effects. Some pathogens are unique to HIV disease, and others that cause mild or self-limiting disease in immunocompetent hosts may cause severe and prolonged disease in the setting of advanced HIV infection. A careful history may provide important diagnostic clues as to the possible cause of diarrhea.[6] The patient's most recent and nadir CD4 count, history of opportunistic infections, currently prescribed antiretroviral regimen, and prophylactic antibiotics all help determine the pathogens to which the patient is susceptible.[7,8] The duration, frequency, volume, and character of the diarrhea, as well as associated symptoms such as weight loss, fever, and abdominal pain help to narrow the differential. For example, several weeks of

---

Box 1
Causes of acute diarrhea in HIV

Bacterial infections

- *Salmonella*[a]
- *Shigella*[a]
- *Campylobacter*[a]
- *Yersinia*
- *Escherichia coli*
- *Vibrio*
- *Clostridium difficile*[a]

Viral infections

- Norwalk virus[a]
- Rotavirus[a]
- Adenovirus

Parasitic infections

- *Giardia lamblia*[a]
- *Entamoeba histolytica*[a]
- *Blastocystis hominis*

Antibiotic associated diarrhea

Antiretroviral associated diarrhea[a]

[a] More common causes.

---

voluminous watery diarrhea with cramps, bloating, and nausea in a patient with low CD4 counts would suggest small bowel infection with *Cryptosporidium*, *Microsporidium*, *Isospora belli*, or *Giardia* organisms.[9] Similarly, a recent onset of small-volume diarrhea with hematochezia and tenesmus would raise suspicion for *Shigella* or *Campylobacter* infection of the large bowel, whereas a longer duration of these symptoms would suggest colitis from cytomegalovirus (CMV), herpes, or *Clostridium difficile*.[8] In addition, a complete list of current medications should be obtained, and particular attention given to antiretroviral medications, any recent changes in medications, recent antibiotic use, over-the-counter medications, and medications that decrease gastric acidity (H2 antagonists and proton pump inhibitors).[7] The latter have been shown to increase risk of acquiring *C difficile*. An explicit sexual history should be taken as anal-oral contact increases the risk of certain pathogens.[8]

As with all cases of diarrhea, a complete history should include information about recent travel, dietary changes, pets, water source, sick contacts (especially children), any comorbid conditions, and family history of chronic diarrhea or irritable bowel disease. If the patient is employed in a food-handling industry, health department notification may be required.

Physical examination should focus on the abdominal examination, noting location and amount of tenderness, quality of bowel sounds, stool guaiac examination, and any associated hepatosplenomegaly. The presence of fever and signs of dehydration, such as dry mucous membranes and tachycardia, should be noted (**Box 3**).

Box 2
Causes of persistent and chronic diarrhea in HIV

Bacterial and mycobacterial infections
- *Escherichia coli*
- *Salmonella*
- *Shigella*
- *Campylobacter jejuni*
- *Clostridium difficile*[a]
- Tuberculosis
- *Mycobacterium avium* complex (MAC)[a]

Parasitic infections
- *Cryptosporidium*[a]
- *Microsporidium*[a]
- *Isospora belli*
- *Giardia lamblia*[a]
- *Cyclospora*
- *Entamoeba histolytica*[a]

Viral infections
- Cytomegalovirus
- Herpes
- HIV (AIDS enteropathy)

Other causes
- Kaposi sarcoma
- Lymphomas
- Malabsorption
- Medication side effects[a]
- Small bowel overgrowth
- Functional disorders
- Irritable bowel syndrome
- Pancreatic insufficiency (MAC, cytomegalovirus, pentamidine, didanosine)

[a] More common causes.

Stratifying patients by their most recent CD4 count provides a useful way to identify which patients are at risk for infections unique to HIV and at increased risk of complications from more common pathogens. In patients with relatively intact immune function, as measured by a current CD4 count greater than 200, acute diarrhea should be evaluated in essentially the same way as diarrhea in a patient without HIV. Viral gastroenteritis and HIV medication-related diarrhea account for most cases of diarrhea in this population, but a higher incidence of common enteric pathogens is also seen in this group of patients.[7] With decreasing CD4 counts, other pathogens increasingly predominate, and the prevalence of persistent and chronic diarrhea increases several-fold (see later discussion). Most infections causing persistent and chronic

---

Box 3
Key components of history and examination

History

- HIV status: current CD4 T-cell count, antiretroviral treatment, and history of opportunistic infections
- Duration of symptoms, frequency, characteristics of stool, amount, weight loss
- Medications: including over-the-counter medications, recent change in medication, HIV medication, use of proton pump inhibitors or H2 blockers
- Recent antibiotic use or hospitalization
- Abdominal symptoms or constitutional symptoms
- Travel, food habits, sexual activity
- Pets
- Water source
- Sick contacts, children, day care
- Comorbidities (eg, diabetes, pancreatitis)
- Family history of bowel disease (eg, irritable bowel disease)
- Employment (eg, food service employee)

Examination

- Vital signs, fever, weight
- Signs of dehydration, orthostatic hypotension, tachycardia, dry mucous membranes
- Abdominal examination, tenderness, hepatosplenomegaly
- Skin evidence of rash or Kaposi sarcoma
- Signs of systemic illness

---

diarrhea are seen more frequently in patients with more advanced HIV infection, for example, *Mycobacterium avium* complex (MAC), *Microsporidium*, chronic *Cryptosporidium*, and CMV.[7,10,11]

In addition to the common causes of diarrhea in the normal host, patients with HIV are at higher risk of the following pathologies, based on CD4 count:

CD4 greater than 200

- HIV medication-associated diarrhea
- Self-limiting bacterial AGE
- Viral AGE
- *Giardia*
- *Entamoeba histolytica*
- Self-limiting *Cryptosporidium*
- Tuberculosis
- Small bowel overgrowth

CD4 50 to 200

- All of the above
- Invasive/systemic *Salmonella*
- Invasive bacterial enteritis
- *Clostridium difficile*

CD4 less than 50

- All of the above
- MAC
- Chronic and severe *Cryptosporidium* and *Microsporidium*
- HIV enteropathy
- CMV colitis.

Patients with HIV are often at risk for additional infections because of overlapping risk factors for sexually transmitted infections. Proctitis caused by gonorrhea and *Chlamydia* may be mistaken for colitis. Infections causing enteritis that may be transmitted via a fecal-oral route include *Salmonella, Shigella, Campylobacter jejuni,* hepatitis A, *Yersinia, Giardia lamblia,* and *Entamoeba histolytica* (**Box 4**).

Associated symptoms such as long-standing fever and night sweats may suggest underlying mycobacterial disease, such as MAC or TB.[12] Profound dehydration in a patient with less than 200 CD4 cells may suggest cryptosporidial infection.[9] Patients with CMV colitis may experience odynophagia or visual field defects from concomitant esophageal and retinal CMV infection.

Additional focused examination may be useful depending on the clinical scenario. A patient with CD4 less than 50 and symptoms referable to colitis should have a retinal examination for possible CMV. The presence of a violaceous nodular rash consistent with Kaposi sarcoma or the presence of the white patchy mucosal lesions of oral or vaginal candidiasis suggests a CD4 count less than 200 in a patient whose stage of HIV disease is unknown.

Because patients infected with HIV may receive multiple antibiotics, higher rates of small bowel overgrowth and *C difficile* are reported. The prevalence of small bowel overgrowth in patients infected with HIV may be greater than 30%.[7] Small bowel overgrowth is characterized by excess growth of mostly gram-negative enteric flora, resulting in chronic diarrhea and malabsorption, culminating in malnutrition and vitamin deficiencies.

HIV itself infects the gut wall and can cause a chronic diarrheal illness associated with malabsorption and weight loss. This so-called HIV enteropathy remains poorly defined, and is generally seen in advanced HIV disease (CD4 <100).[1] It is a diagnosis of exclusion.

Box 4
Diarrhea-causing pathogens that may be transmitted sexually

Infections that may be transmitted sexually

- *Shigella*
- *Campylobacter*
- *Yersinia*
- *Giardia*
- *Entamoeba*
- *Cryptosporidium*
- Hepatitis A
- Herpes simplex
- Gonorrhea
- *Chlamydia*

The most common noninfectious causes of diarrhea in patients infected with HIV are medication side effects, particularly the protease inhibitors, which are the backbone of many potent antiretroviral regimens (**Box 5**). Patients report a temporal association with initiation of the medication, and generally report moderate- to low-volume watery diarrhea or loose stools, possibly with abdominal bloating, gas, and discomfort. Abdominal cramps, fever, bloody stool, and dehydration are absent. The diarrhea may wane after 4 to 6 weeks on the medication, but often persists, particularly with nelfinavir, ritonavir, and lopinavir.[1,13] Other noninfectious causes include infiltrative diseases such as gastrointestinal Kaposi sarcoma and non-Hodgkin lymphoma. Up to 15% of patients with visceral Kaposi sarcoma do not have skin involvement.

Because of the broad range of possible enteric pathogens requiring distinct treatments, particularly in patients with advanced HIV disease, microbiologic diagnosis should always be pursued.[1,14,15] Depending on the clinical scenario, the following investigations may be appropriate:

- Stool culture and sensitivity
  ○ Specify cultures for *E coli* 0157, *Vibrio*, *Yersina* if diarrhea is bloody or patient systemically ill
- Stool ova and parasite examination
  ○ *Microsporidia* is ordered separately
- *Giardia* antigen test
- *C difficile* toxin assay
- Stool for white blood cell counts, red blood cell counts, fecal fat, Na and K for osmotic gap
- Endoscopy: sigmoidoscopy, colonoscopy ± terminal ileum aspirate, esophago-gastroduodenoscopy

---

Box 5
Commonly used HIV-related medications that can cause diarrhea

HIV protease inhibitors

- Amprenavir (Agenerase)
- Darunavir (Prezista)
- Fosamprenavir (Lexiva)
- Lopinavir (Kaletra)
- Nelfinavir (Viracept)
- Ritonavir (Norvir)
- Saquinavir (Fortovase)
- Tipranavir (Aptivus)

HIV nucleoside reverse transcriptase inhibitors

- Abacavir (Ziagen)
- Didanosine (Videx)
- Stavudine (Zerit)
- Tenofovir (Viread)

Antibiotics

- Clindamycin
- Trimethoprim/sulfamethoxazole

- Radiology: plain film for free air (perforation), thumb printing, computed tomography scan of the abdomen.

Although certain pathogens require upper or lower endoscopy with mucosal aspirate cultures and/or biopsy for diagnosis, it is reasonable to initiate a step-wise approach in the emergency department. Initial evaluation should include stool culture and sensitivity and examination for ova and parasites (O&P).[16] Because of the relatively low sensitivity of only 1 O&P examination (~50%), patients should have follow-up O&P examination on a second and third stool sample after discharge. If the CD4 count is less than 200, examinations for *Microsporidium* and *Cryptosporidium* should also be specifically requested with the O&P examination.[16] A history of recent antibiotic therapy or hospital admission should prompt stool collection for *C difficile* toxin assay, although this study should be considered even in patients without these risk factors. Fecal leukocytes may support a diagnosis of bacterial gastroenteritis, but their absence does not rule out infection in a patient infected with HIV, and this is generally not a useful test in this population. All febrile patients should receive blood cultures to rule out bacteremia from *Salmonella* or other enteric bacteria, and separate mycobacterial blood culture should be sent in febrile patients with CD4 less than 100 to rule out MAC.[6]

Patients with persistent or chronic diarrhea in whom this initial workup has not revealed a cause should be referred for endoscopic evaluation, and a noninfectious cause, such as medication side effect or irritable bowel syndrome, should be considered.[13,17] Colonoscopy or sigmoidoscopy with mucosal biopsy is generally required for diagnosis of CMV colitis.[18] Diagnosis of MAC is usually made by mycobacterial blood culture, although it may only appear in mucosal aspirate.[16,17] Other diagnoses that may require upper or lower endoscopy with biopsy and/or microbiologic examination of mucosal aspirate include *Microsporidium* and *Cryptosporidium*.[17] The diagnostic value of radiographic studies in evaluating diarrhea is very low compared with endoscopy, and these are not generally indicated.

MANAGEMENT

In patients with CD4 counts greater than 200, most cases of acute diarrhea are self-limiting infections that can be managed conservatively with oral rehydration, symptomatic treatment, and dietary modifications, with early follow-up for results of stool studies. Patients with CD4 less than 200, febrile, evidence of systemic involvement, and requiring admission for other reasons may be empirically treated once appropriate specimens have been obtained for examination and culture.

When the cause of diarrhea has already been established by microbiologic or other means, antimicrobial therapy should be tailored to the specific pathogen (**Table 2**). Empiric therapy should be directed at common gram-negative enteric pathogens (eg, *Salmonella*, *Shigella*, *Yersinia*, *Campylobacter*, and so forth). A quinolone, such as ciprofloxacin 500 mg twice a day or levofloxacin 500 mg every day for 5 days is recommended. If clinical suspicion for a parasitic infection, such as *Giardia* or *Entamoeba histolytica* is high, metronidazole 250 mg to 750 mg three times a day or tinidazole 2 g daily can be substituted.

Patients presenting to the emergency department with persistent or chronic diarrhea despite treatment of enteric bacteria may be empirically treated with metronidazole or tinidazole for parasites, and cipro/flagyl for bacterial overgrowth. If 3 stool O&Ps are negative and their symptoms are more consistent with an infectious cause than a medication side effect or irritable bowel syndrome, these patients should be

Table 2
Clinical features and treatment of common diarrhea-causing pathogens

Organism	Clinical Features	Treatment
Salmonella	May be septic and invasive in low CD4; usually food acquired	Ciprofloxacin 500–750 twice a day for 14 days, or intravenous ceftriaxone; if CD4 <200, treat for 4–6 weeks
Campylobacter	Possible sexual exposure; may also be invasive (bloody, fever) with bacteremia/ extraintestinal in CD4 <200	Ciprofloxacin 500 twice a day for 3–5 days (2 weeks if bacteremic) or azithromycin 500 every day for 3–5 days (some quinolone resistance)
Shigella	Possible sexual exposure; may be bloody, with fever and upper gastrointestinal symptoms	Ciprofloxicin 500 twice a day for 3–5 days
Giardia	Gas, bloating, cramps, foul smelling stools	Metronidazole 250–500 3 times a day for 7 days or tinidazole 2 g single dose
Isospora	Watery, afebrile	Trimethoprim/sulfamethoxazole double strength 4 times a day for 10 days
E histolytica	Gas, bloating, cramps, foul smelling stools, may be bloody	Metronidazole 750 3 times a day for 10 days or tinidazole 2 g every day for 3–5 days
MAC	Occurs exclusively in low CD4; fever, weight loss, anemia, night sweats, hepatomegaly, increased alkaline phosphatase level	Clarithromycin 500 twice a day + ethambutol 20 mg/kg/ d indefinitely, and antiretroviral therapy
C difficile	Previous antibiotics or hospitalization	Metronidazole 500 3 times a day for 10 days
Cryptosporidium	Large volumes, nausea/ vomiting, cramps, electrolyte imbalance, acidosis in low CD4	Immunocompetent: nitazoxanide 500 twice a day for 3–5 days CD4 <100: nitazoxanide 500 twice a day or paromomycin 1 g twice a day + azithromycin 600 every day; + antiretroviral therapy
Microsporidium	Watery stools, malabsorption; fever uncommon	Albendazole 400–800 twice a day for 2–4 weeks
CMV	Occurs exclusively in CD4 <50; colitis, lower abdominal pain, bright red blood per rectum; may coexist with retinitis; requires biopsy for diagnosis	Ganciclovir 5 mg/kg intravenously twice a day and antiretroviral therapy

referred for endoscopy. Irritable bowel syndrome and transient lactose intolerance can follow an acute bacterial gastroenteritis. Local health departments may require notification of positive culture results for certain pathogens (eg, *Shigella*, gonorrhea, and so forth), and sexual partner notification may be warranted.

Dietary modification may assist in ameliorating diarrhea in all patients. Recommended foods include complex carbohydrates in the form of boiled starches and cereals, such as potatoes, noodles, rice, wheat, and oats, with salt, along with boiled vegetables and lean meats. Soups, crackers, yogurt, and bananas are often eaten. Lactose-containing foods and high-fat foods should be avoided. Symptomatic treatment of patients with chronic diarrhea and in select afebrile patients with acute nonbloody diarrhea is recommended. Typically loperamide (4 mg initially, then 2 mg after each unformed stool) or diphenoxylate (4 mg four times a day) are used.[7] Bulking agents such as psyllium are often beneficial. Patients with advanced HIV disease and infections such as Cryptosporidium or MAC may experience severe chronic diarrhea causing dehydration, malnutrition, and weight loss. In these patients, a more aggressive attempt at slowing intestinal motility can include oral tincture of opium or subcutaneous administration of octreotide.[19] In all patients with dehydration, oral rehydration solutions provide more effective rehydration than sports drinks, and are less likely to cause hypernatremia than high-sodium foods such as chicken soup. Intravenous rehydration is indicated for all patients with moderate to severe dehydration. Although antiretroviral medications undoubtedly contribute to diarrhea in patients with infectious causes, many of these infections are incurable without sustained treatment of HIV and immune restoration. Antiretroviral medications should be discontinued only as a last resort and in consultation with the prescribing practitioner as any changes may affect disease resistance patterns and future treatment options.

Patients infected with HIV with lower CD4 counts are at higher risk of *Salmonella* bacteremia and septicemia. Complications of *Salmonella* bacteremia in this population include septicemia, pyelonephritis, intraabdominal abscesses, osteomyelitis, and septic arthritis. Patients with suspected or known *Salmonella* bacteremia should be admitted for treatment with intravenous quinolone, and for further workup and observation. Patients with CD4 counts less than 200 and *Salmonella* bacteremia should be treated for 4 to 6 weeks, and if relapse occurs, should be maintained indefinitely on a suppressive fluroquinolone therapy, such as ciprofloxacin.[8,20]

Patients with advanced HIV and opportunistic enteric infections (particularly *Cryptosporidium*) can have massive volume loss resulting in hemodynamic compromise, significant electrolyte imbalance (especially hypokalemia), and refractory acidosis from loss of bicarbonate. Such patients require admission for aggressive intravenous rehydration, electrolyte repletion, antimotility agents, and correction of acidosis.

Patients with low CD4 counts and chronic diarrhea from conditions such as MAC, *Microsporidium*, *Cryptosporidium* or HIV enteropathy can develop nutritional, caloric, and vitamin deficiencies. In concert with the catabolic state often seen in advanced HIV, this can result in a state resembling starvation that, in its severe form, requires admission. Rarely, patients with extensive gastrointestinal Kaposi sarcoma can experience gastrointestinal hemorrhage. Severe infectious colitis (eg, *C difficile*) or infiltrative processes (eg, lymphoma) can cause perforation.

Admission to the hospital should be considered in any patient with CD4 less than 200 cells/mm^3 and in patients with hepatosplenomegaly on examination, and is recommended for patients with the following features:

- CD4 less than 200 who have fever and/or signs or symptoms of systemic involvement
- Known or suspected bacteremia
- CD4 less than 200 and known *Salmonella* infection
- Severe dehydration, acidosis, or electrolyte imbalance.

All patients should be referred for rapid follow-up of initial stool studies and blood cultures, and patients with persistent symptoms and negative stool studies should be referred for endoscopy.

Universal blood and bodily fluid precautions are sufficient infection control methods for most pathogens associated with diarrhea in patients with HIV. When caring for patients with known *C difficile* infection, use only soap and water for hand hygiene, as alcohol-based hand rubs may not be as effective against spore-forming bacteria. Place these patients in private rooms, if available, use gloves during patient care, and dedicated equipment whenever possible.

SUMMARY

Diarrhea is common in patients infected with HIV, and is associated with a range of common causes and opportunistic infections. The diagnostic strategy involves discerning acute from chronic diarrhea, and small bowel pathology from large bowel involvement, followed by opportunistic infection risk stratification based on CD4 count. Patients without advanced immunosuppression are most likely suffering from common viral and bacterial causes and medication side effects, whereas the differential diagnosis for those with CD4 less than 200 is much broader. These immunosuppressed patients often require inpatient workup and management, as do patients with systemic symptoms, severe dehydration, acidosis, and electrolyte imbalance. An attempt at definitive microbiologic diagnosis should be made for most patients, particularly those with low CD4 counts and with chronic diarrhea, but initial therapy is usually empiric.

REFERENCES

1. Call SA, Heudebert G, Saag M, et al. The changing etiology of chronic diarrhea in HIV-infected patients with CD4 cell counts less than 200 cells/mm^3. Am J Gastroenterol 2000;95(11):3142–6.
2. Weber R, Ledergerber B, Zbinden R, et al. Enteric infections and diarrhea in human immunodeficiency virus-infected persons: prospective community-based cohort study. Swiss HIV Cohort Study. Arch Intern Med 1999;159(13):1473–80.
3. Crotty B, Smallwood RA. Investigating diarrhea in patients with acquired immunodeficiency syndrome. Gastroenterology 1996;110(1):296–8.
4. Yoshida D, Caruso JM. Abdominal pain in the HIV infected patient. J Emerg Med 2002;23(2):111–6.
5. Sharpstone D, Gazzard B. Gastrointestinal manifestations of HIV infection. Lancet 1996;348(9024):379–83.
6. Mayer HB, Wanke CA. Diagnostic strategies in HIV-infected patients with diarrhea. AIDS 1994;8(12):1639–48.
7. Morpeth SC, Thielman NM. Diarrhea in patients with AIDS. Curr Treat Options Gastroenterol 2006;9(1):23–37.
8. Angulo FJ, Swerdlow DL. Bacterial enteric infections in persons infected with human immunodeficiency virus. Clin Infect Dis 1995;21(Suppl 1):S84–93.
9. Chen XM, Keithly JS, Paya CV, et al. Cryptosporidiosis. N Engl J Med 2002;346(22):1723–31.
10. Cohen J, West AB, Bini EJ. Infectious diarrhea in human immunodeficiency virus. Gastroenterol Clin North Am 2001;30(3):637–64.
11. Asmuth DM, DeGirolami PC, Federman M, et al. Clinical features of microsporidiosis in patients with AIDS. Clin Infect Dis 1994;18(5):819–25.

12. Wilcox CM. Chronic unexplained diarrhea in AIDS: approach to diagnosis and management. AIDS Patient Care STDS 1997;11(1):13–7.
13. Guest JL, Ruffin C, Tschampa JM, et al. Differences in rates of diarrhea in patients with human immunodeficiency virus receiving lopinavir-ritonavir or nelfinavir. Pharmacotherapy 2004;24(6):727–35.
14. Blanshard C, Francis N, Gazzard BG. Investigation of chronic diarrhoea in acquired immunodeficiency syndrome. A prospective study of 155 patients. Gut 1996;39(6):824–32.
15. Wilcox CM, Schwartz DA, Cotsonis G, et al. Chronic unexplained diarrhea in human immunodeficiency virus infection: determination of the best diagnostic approach. Gastroenterology 1996;110(1):30–7.
16. Greenberg PD, Koch J, Cello JP. Diagnosis of *Cryptosporidium parvum* in patients with severe diarrhea and AIDS. Dig Dis Sci 1996;41(11):2286–90.
17. Kearney DJ, Steuerwald M, Koch J, et al. A prospective study of endoscopy in HIV-associated diarrhea. Am J Gastroenterol 1999;94(3):596–602.
18. Dieterich DT, Rahmin M. Cytomegalovirus colitis in AIDS: presentation in 44 patients and a review of the literature. J Acquir Immune Defic Syndr 1991;4(Suppl 1):S29–35.
19. Simon DM, Cello JP, Valenzuela J, et al. Multicenter trial of octreotide in patients with refractory acquired immunodeficiency syndrome-associated diarrhea. Gastroenterology 1995;108(6):1753–60.
20. Nelson MR, Shanson DC, Hawkins DA, et al. *Salmonella, Campylobacter* and *Shigella* in HIV-seropositive patients. AIDS 1992;6(12):1495–8.

Altered Mental Status in HIV-Infected Patients

Emily L. Ho, MD, PhD[a,b,*], Cheryl A. Jay, MD[a,b,c]

KEYWORDS

- Human immunodeficiency virus • AIDS • Altered mental status
- Central nervous system infection

Human immunodeficiency virus (HIV)-infected patients are vulnerable to developing altered mental status (AMS) for myriad reasons including: the effects of HIV itself, the accompanying immune dysfunction, associated systemic illness, comorbid psychiatric disorders, and complicated medication regimens.[1,2] Combination antiretroviral therapy (ART) has decreased the incidence of central nervous system (CNS) opportunistic infections (OIs) and HIV-associated dementia, but the benefits are not absolute.[3] Moreover, patients with undiagnosed or untreated HIV infection may present with AMS. In addition to CNS OIs and complications of complex multisystem disease, immune reconstitution events developing in the early weeks and months after initiating ART may affect the brain and cause AMS.[4]

EPIDEMIOLOGY

Before ART became the standard of HIV care in high-income countries, approximately half of HIV-infected patients developed symptomatic central or peripheral nervous system disease, with neuropathology observed in nearly all individuals dying with HIV/acquired immunodeficiency syndrome (AIDS).[5,6] Since the advent of ART, the incidence of dementia, the major cerebral OIs (cryptococcal meningitis, toxoplasmosis, progressive multifocal leukoencephalopathy [PML]), and primary CNS lymphoma (PCNSL) has fallen.[3,7,8] HIV-associated dementia is also less common and more indolent in patients on ART.[3,9] In the United States, fewer patients now

Funding support: Emily L. Ho has received a Clinical Research Training Fellowship from the American Academy of Neurology.

[a] Department of Neurology, University of California San Francisco, San Francisco, CA, USA
[b] Department of Neurology, 4M62, San Francisco General Hospital, 1001 Potrero Avenue, San Francisco, CA 94110, USA
[c] Positive Health Program, San Francisco General Hospital, 1001 Potrero Avenue, San Francisco, CA 94110, USA
* Corresponding author. Department of Neurology, 4M62, San Francisco General Hospital, 1001 Potrero Avenue, San Francisco, CA 94110.
E-mail address: Emily.Ho@ucsf.edu

Emerg Med Clin N Am 28 (2010) 311–323
doi:10.1016/j.emc.2010.01.012
0733-8627/10/$ – see front matter © 2010 Elsevier Inc. All rights reserved.

develop the mutism, quadriparesis, and incontinence that were common with late-stage infection in the early years of the AIDS epidemic.

In approximately 25% of patients, the first weeks and months after initiation of ART may be complicated by the immune reconstitution inflammatory syndrome (IRIS), with paradoxic worsening of previously diagnosed or subclinical OIs or the development of autoimmune disorders.[10] IRIS affects most organ systems, including the brain. Patients with tuberculosis may be at particular risk of IRIS, and tuberculous meningitis and tuberculoma associated with initiation of ART have been reported. Clinical exacerbation of cryptococcal meningitis, worsening PML, and rapidly progressive dementia in the setting of immune reconstitution has also been described.[4] The clinical spectrum of IRIS is not yet fully defined, and should be considered when patients develop AMS in the first weeks and months after starting ART.

Patients with HIV are at increased risk for substance abuse, affective disorders, and psychosis.[2] Injection drug users with HIV remain at risk for the neurologic sequelae of endocarditis, including brain abscess, meningitis, ischemic stroke from septic embolism, and hemorrhagic stroke from mycotic aneurysm rupture. Patients coinfected with hepatitis C are at risk for cognitive impairment even in the absence of cirrhosis and portal hypertension.[11] In addition, HIV-infected patients who use cocaine or methamphetamine are at risk for seizures and ischemic and hemorrhagic stroke.

Medications used to treat HIV disease or associated conditions may also contribute to AMS. Antiretroviral agents, particularly the nonnucleoside reverse transcriptase inhibitor (NNRTI) efavirenz, can cause cerebral side effects, including psychiatric syndromes, as can the myriad other drugs used to treat HIV/AIDS and comorbid medical conditions.[2]

Finally, as a multisystem illness, HIV infection can cause AMS even without primary neurologic, psychiatric, or medication-associated illness. For example, patients with HIV-associated nephropathy are subject to the neurologic complications of uremia, including encephalopathy. Septic patients may present with AMS in the absence of CNS infection.

CLINICAL FEATURES

As for any patient presenting to the emergency department (ED) with AMS, important elements of the history include the temporal progression of symptoms, drug use (prescription, over-the-counter, illicit), trauma, focal symptoms (aphasia, neglect, hemianopsia, hemiparesis, hemisensory loss), seizures, and symptoms suggesting increased intracranial pressure (ICP) (**Box 1** and **Table 1**). Additional important details in the HIV-infected patient include recent and nadir CD4 count, viral load and, for patients on ART, the specific regimen and the duration of therapy. Regardless of treatment history, patients with CD4 counts less than 200 cells/mm^3 are at highest risk for cerebral OIs, primary CNS lymphoma, and HIV-associated dementia.[1,3,5,8,9] Patients with prior cerebral toxoplasmosis or cryptococcal meningitis require secondary prophylaxis unless ART increases the CD4 count to greater than 200 cells/mm^3 for 6 months.[7] Clinicians should have a high index of suspicion for relapse in an altered patient with a history of cerebral OIs.

For patients recently started on ART, additional diagnostic considerations include medication side effects (eg, efavirenz) or IRIS.[2,4,9,10] Patients with CD4 counts of more than 200 cells/mm^3 may be at risk for the major HIV-related brain disorders if treatment was begun within the past 6 months or if there is evidence of treatment failure, such as falling CD4 count, rising viral load, or both.

It is important to remember that the immune dysfunction that predisposes HIV-infected patients to cerebral infections also masks the signs and symptoms

---

Box 1
Key elements of the history

- Temporal progression of symptoms
- Drug use (prescription, nonprescription, illicit)
- Trauma
- Focal symptoms (aphasia, neglect, hemianopsia, hemiparesis, hemisensory deficit)
- Seizures
- Symptoms suggesting increased ICP such as progressive or morning headache, nausea and vomiting, or deteriorating level of consciousness

Additional important details in the HIV-infected patient include:

- Recent and nadir CD4 count
- Viral load
- Specific antiretroviral regimen and the duration of therapy

---

associated with similar disorders in immunocompetent individuals. In particular, the absence of fever or headache should not be used to exclude CNS infection, nor should the absence of meningismus be used to exclude meningitis (**Box 2**). Neurologic examination should focus on identifying evidence of increased ICP (anisocoria, papilledema) or focal cerebral dysfunction, such as visual field deficits,

Table 1
Differential diagnosis of AMS in the HIV high-risk population

IDU	• Drug intoxication or withdrawal • Endocarditis with septic encephalopathy • Ischemic stroke from septic embolism • Hemorrhagic stroke from mycotic aneurysm rupture • Brain abscess and/or meningitis
Cocaine and methamphetamine	• Seizure • Ischemic or hemorrhagic stroke
Medications	Prescription: • Efavirenz • Psychotropic drugs • Opiates and other analgesics Nonprescription: • Antihistamines • Ethanol (intoxication or withdrawal) Illicit: • Heroin • Stimulants • Other drugs of abuse
Multisystem disease	• Uremic encephalopathy • Hepatic encephalopathy • Electrolyte abnormalities
Focal cerebral dysfunction	See **Table 2**
Diffuse cerebral dysfunction	See **Table 3**

Abbreviation: IDU, injection drug user.

> **Box 2**
> **Key points in recognizing subtle CNS infections in advanced HIV disease**
>
> - Absence of fever or headache does not exclude cerebral infections.
> - Absence of meningismus does not exclude meningitis.
> - Neurologic examination should focus on identifying increased ICP and focal cerebral dysfunction.

lateralized motor (pronator drift, hemiparesis, reflex asymmetry, unilateral Babinski sign) or sensory deficits and, in patients alert enough to walk, gait disorder.

Determining whether the patient's AMS appears to be a manifestation of focal or diffuse cerebral dysfunction helps focus the long list of diagnostic considerations.

DIFFERENTIAL DIAGNOSIS
Focal Cerebral Dysfunction

Patients with signs or symptoms suggesting lateralized brain disturbance (**Table 2**) may have AMS by several mechanisms, more than one of which can coexist in a given patient. Brainstem or cerebellar lesions may impair level of alertness early. Patients with solitary hemispheric lesions are awake unless there is significant mass effect, concomitant meningitis, or toxic-metabolic encephalopathy. Dominant hemisphere lesions cause aphasia (often with associated right homonymous hemianopsia, hemiparesis, or hemisensory loss) and nondominant hemisphere processes cause neglect or inattention with left-sided visual, motor, or sensory dysfunction. Patients with old focal brain lesions, such as prior trauma, stroke, tumor, or infection, may experience a worsening of stable focal deficits in the setting of drug intoxication, metabolic derangement, meningitis, or seizure. In general, CNS OIs and primary CNS lymphoma are more common in patients with CD4 counts less than 200 cells/mm^3, whereas cerebrovascular disease (which may complicate CNS infection, particularly tuberculosis [TB] or syphilitic meningitis) is more common in HIV-infected patients with focal cerebral deficit at higher CD4 counts.[12]

Diffuse Cerebral Dysfunction

Patients with a depressed level of alertness or milder cognitive or behavioral disturbances without aphasia, neglect, or lateralizing motor, reflex, or sensory findings may have multiple brain lesions, meningitis, delirium, psychiatric decompensation, or have had an unwitnessed seizure (**Table 3**). Dementia is a risk factor for delirium, but dementia alone does not cause a depressed level of alertness (lethargy, obtundation, or stupor) except in its very advanced stages.

Additional considerations in patients with CNS infection or lymphoma who decompensate include medication effects and electrolyte disorder, particularly hyponatremia from the syndrome of inappropriate antidiuretic hormone secretion or cerebral salt wasting, or hypernatremia from diabetes insipidus.

LABORATORY AND RADIOGRAPHIC FINDINGS

Initial evaluation proceeds as for any patient with AMS, with particular attention to evidence of increased ICP, first-time seizure, trauma, or focal cerebral deficit (**Table 4**). Appropriate laboratory studies include electrolytes, blood urea nitrogen

Table 2
Clinical features: focal cerebral dysfunction in HIV/AIDS

Common Etiologies (usually CD4 <200 cells/mm^3)	
Cerebral toxoplasmosis	• Altered mental status, focal cerebral symptoms, or seizure, usually evolving over days to weeks, often with fever and headache • Reactivation of previously acquired, often asymptomatic, infection with the parasite *Toxoplasma gondii* • Unusual in patients on trimethoprim-sulfamethoxazole for *Pneumocystis* prophylaxis, because the drug also provides primary prophylaxis against toxoplasmosis
Progressive multifocal leukoencephalopathy (PML)	• Focal deficit, often homonymous hemianopsia or hemiparesis, steadily progressive over months without headache or fever • Reactivation of previously acquired, often asymptomatic, infection with the JC virus
Primary CNS lymphoma (PCNSL)	• Gradually progressive focal deficit or cognitive dysfunction, sometimes with headache, evolving over months • Almost always associated with EBV in tumor cells in HIV-infected patients
Less Common Infectious Causes	
CMV ventriculoencephalitis	• CD4 count <100 cells/mm^3 • Cognitive impairment with brainstem findings (cranial neuropathies, ataxia) • Sometimes associated with polyradiculitis (cauda equina syndrome with paraparesis, incontinence, and hyporeflexia) evolving over days to weeks • CSF profile may resemble bacterial meningitis with elevated protein, polymorphonuclear pleocytosis, and low or normal glucose
Brain abscess (bacterial or fungal)	• Progressive focal cerebral deficit, with or without headache • Consider in patients with proven or suspected bacteremia (injection drug use, indwelling line, chronic skin infection, prosthetic heart valve) or craniofacial infection • Consider angioinvasive fungi (*Mucor* or *Aspergillus*, discussed below) in patients with CD4 count <50 cells/mm^3 and associated sinus infection
Tuberculoma	• Presentation similar to brain abscess • Rare, but may develop as immune reconstitution inflammatory syndrome in patients on antituberculous therapy for systemic TB (or tuberculous meningitis) in the first weeks to months of ART
Stroke	
Meningovascular syphilis	• Occurs with or after secondary syphilis as ischemic stroke(s) with or without clinically manifested meningitis
Angioinvasive fungi (*Aspergillus, Mucor*)	• CD4 count <50 cells/mm^3, associated sinus infection or palatal lesion or brain abscess, in addition to hemorrhagic or ischemic stroke(s)
VZV vasculopathy	• Multiple small-vessel strokes with recent or remote history of shingles
Bacterial endocarditis	• Septic embolism (infarction, abscess, or both), mycotic aneurysm rupture, bacterial meningitis

Abbreviations: CSF, cerebrospinal fluid; CMV, cytomegalovirus; EBV, Epstein-Barr virus; TB, tuberculosis; VZV, varicella-zoster virus.

Table 3
Clinical features: diffuse cerebral dysfunction in HIV/AIDS

Common Etiologies (usually CD4 <200 cells/mm^3)

HIV-associated dementia	• Cognitive, behavioral, and motor slowing over months with hyperreflexia and, in more advanced disease, gait disturbance • More common in patients with untreated HIV disease • Alertness is typically preserved except in end-stage dementia or if there is a coexisting cause for altered mental status
Cryptococcal meningitis	• Most common complaint is mild to moderate headache • Some patients present with symptomatic increased intracranial pressure, including coma • Severe headache with prominent meningismus is unusual, except as a manifestation of immune reconstitution inflammatory syndrome

Other Causes of Meningitis

Tuberculous meningitis	• Usually presents as chronic meningitis with typical symptoms (headache, meningismus, altered mental status, cranial neuropathies), sometimes with small-vessel ischemic stroke • Risk of extrapulmonary disease, including meningitis or tuberculoma, is increased in HIV-positive patients • May present as immune reconstitution event in patients with systemic TB or as exacerbation of TB meningitis (in the first weeks to months of ART)
Syphilitic meningitis	• Occurs weeks to years after primary infection, usually as an aseptic or chronic meningitis with or without cranial neuropathies • May be complicated by ischemic stroke (meningovascular syphilis), seizures, or hydrocephalus
Lymphomatous meningitis	• Presents as headache, altered mental status, cranial neuropathies, or cauda equina syndrome, individually or in combination • Usually with history of systemic lymphoma, although may occasionally be presenting feature
Bacterial meningitis	• Consider *Listeria monocytogenes*, in addition to *Pneumococcus* and *Meningococcus*
Multifocal brain disease	• Toxoplasmosis and PCNSL may occasionally present as diffuse brain dysfunction
Drug ingestion	• Prescription: efavirenz, psychotropic drugs, opiates and other analgesics, among many others • Nonprescription: antihistamines, ethanol • Illicit: heroin, stimulants, and other drugs of abuse
Metabolic encephalopathies	• Renal or hepatic failure, electrolyte abnormalities (in particular sodium, calcium), hypo- or hyperglycemia, hypothyroidism, B$_{12}$ deficiency

(BUN) and creatinine, liver function tests, complete blood count (CBC), prothrombin time, and toxicology screen.

Although magnetic resonance imaging (MRI) is more sensitive for many HIV-related cerebral disorders, multidetector computed tomographic (CT) scanners are preferable for agitated and otherwise unstable patients. If there are contraindications to iodinated

Table 4
Selected HIV-related brain disorders: neuroimaging, CSF

Disorder	Findings
Cerebral toxoplasmosis	• Toxoplasma IgG positive: serologic screening is part of routine HIV care, so results may be available in the medical record of patients with an established HIV diagnosis • CT/MRI (see **Fig. 1**): ring-enhancing lesions with marked surrounding edema in basal ganglia or cortical/subcortical junction • Enhancing lesions with negative *Toxoplasma* serology are more likely to be other infectious cause or primary CNS lymphoma • LP may be contraindicated, depending on imaging results: elevated protein, normal glucose, lymphocytic/monocytic pleocytosis; *Toxoplasma* antibodies usually not done routinely in CSF
PCNSL	• CT/MRI (see **Fig. 2**): Homogeneously enhancing lesion or lesions in periventricular regions or corpus callosum, with mild to moderate surrounding edema • LP may be contraindicated, depending on imaging results: elevated protein, normal glucose (unless associated lymphomatous meningitis, in which case glucose may be low), lymphocytic pleocytosis, sometimes with positive EBV PCR or more rarely cytology
PML	• CT/MRI (see **Fig. 3**): Nonenhancing, asymmetric white matter lesion or lesions, often in parietal or occipital white matter, without surrounding edema in most patients. May be confused with ischemic stroke—sparing of gray matter in PML is a helpful clue • Patients who have just started ART and have IRIS may have atypical imaging findings of enhancement and mass effect • LP: elevated protein, normal glucose, mild lymphocytic pleocytosis, positive JC virus PCR
Cryptococcal meningitis	• CT/MRI: normal (or generalized atrophy) or may show hydrocephalus, gelatinous pseudocysts, or cerebral edema. • LP: elevated opening pressure, normal or elevated protein, normal or low glucose, lymphocytic pleocytosis, positive cryptococcal antigen, positive India ink smear
HIV-associated dementia	• CT/MRI: generalized atrophy with mild, symmetric periventricular white matter abnormalities especially bifrontally • LP: normal opening pressure, normal or elevated protein (<100 mg/dL), normal glucose, mild lymphocytic pleocytosis
Tuberculous meningitis	• CT/MRI: normal or basilar enhancement, hydrocephalus or small-vessel infarctions • LP: elevated opening pressure, elevated protein, low glucose, lymphocytic pleocytosis; negative AFB smear does not exclude diagnosis and cultures are not always positive
Syphilitic meningitis	• CT/MRI: normal or basilar enhancement, sometimes with infarction (meningovascular syphilis) • LP: normal or elevated opening pressure, elevated protein, normal or low glucose, lymphocytic pleocytosis; CSF VDRL is ≤70% sensitive, so diagnosis may depend on positive serum serology with compatible CSF profile and overall clinical picture
CMV ventriculoencephalitis	• CT/MRI: normal or periventricular enhancement, with or without hydrocephalus • LP: may resemble bacterial meningitis with elevated protein, polymorphonuclear pleocytosis, and low or normal glucose, positive CMV PCR

Abbreviations: AFB, acid-fast bacillus; CT, computed tomography; LP, lumbar puncture; MRI, magnetic resonance imaging; PCR, polymerase chain reaction; VDRL, Venereal Disease Research Laboratory test.

contrast, noncontrast CT can identify hydrocephalus, hemorrhage, or large mass lesions that would contraindicate lumbar puncture (LP).

Studies of the yield of noncontrast CT in HIV-infected patients presenting to the ED with neurologic dysfunction indicate that AMS was significantly associated with abnormal findings on CT.[13] For patients with CD4 count less than 200 cells/mm^3, who are at highest risk for HIV-related cerebral complications, CT with and without contrast can sometimes obviate the need for LP if the findings suggest toxoplasmosis (**Fig. 1**), primary CNS lymphoma (**Fig. 2**), or PML (**Fig. 3**).

Whereas neuroradiologic findings in PML are relatively distinct, toxoplasmosis and primary CNS lymphoma can be difficult to distinguish definitively, even by MRI.[14] In patients with meningitis, CT may reveal complications such as edema, infarction, or obstructive or communicating hydrocephalus. Patients with mass lesions should have serum *Toxoplasma* IgG antibodies sent, because a negative serology significantly decreases the likelihood that mass lesions are due to *Toxoplasma gondii*.[1,7,9]

If laboratory studies have not revealed the cause of the patient's AMS and CT reveals no contraindication to LP, cerebrospinal fluid (CSF) examination should be performed. Once the opening pressure is determined, CSF should be withdrawn and sent for protein, glucose, cell count, cryptococcal antigen, and VDRL (Venereal Disease Research Laboratory) test, as well as for bacterial, fungal, and acid-fast bacillus (AFB) smears and cultures. The yield of AFB testing is higher with larger volumes of CSF sent for analysis. If possible, additional CSF should be obtained and held in the laboratory for possible polymerase chain reaction (PCR) testing for JC virus (PML), Epstein-Barr Virus (primary CNS lymphoma), or herpesviruses (cytomegalovirus [CMV], varicella-zoster virus [VZV], herpes simplex virus).

The CSF opening pressure is critical for the management of cryptococcal meningitis, because increased ICP (>200 mm H$_2$O) contributes independently to the morbidity and mortality associated with the infection.[7,8,15] Markedly elevated ICP may require serial LPs, lumbar drainage, or ventriculoperitoneal shunting; measurement of initial opening pressure at the time of admission is very helpful in guiding subsequent management. Acetazolamide and steroids do not have a role in ICP management in HIV-associated cryptococcal meningitis.[7,15]

CSF cryptococcal antigen is very informative because the sensitivity exceeds 95%.[1,7–9] India ink smear is specific, but not as sensitive, and cultures may take weeks

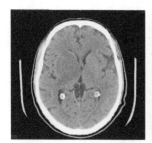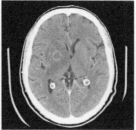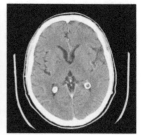

Fig. 1. Cerebral toxoplasmosis. Head CT pre- (*left*) and postcontrast (*center*) from a patient who presented with headache, speech difficulty, and left arm weakness demonstrated a ring-enhancing lesion with surrounding edema in the right globus pallidus (and a smaller lesion in the left temporal lobe not seen on this image). HIV serology came back positive, with positive *Toxoplasma* IgG. The patient's headache and focal deficits resolved with empirical therapy for toxoplasmosis. Repeat postcontrast head CT 2 months later (*right*) showed decreased edema and resolution of abnormal enhancement.

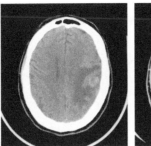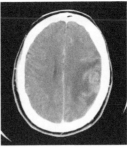

Fig. 2. Primary CNS lymphoma. Head CT pre- (*left*) and postcontrast (*right*) from an untreated AIDS patient who presented with a generalized seizure after a week of dysarthria and right-sided weakness and numbness demonstrated an intrinsically hyperdense left frontoparietal lesion with mass effect and slight homogeneous enhancement. *Toxoplasma* serology was negative, and brain biopsy revealed primary CNS lymphoma.

or months to grow the organism. Similar considerations apply in tuberculous meningitis; hence a negative CSF AFB smear or prior negative CSF culture does not exclude the diagnosis. Typical CSF findings of chronic meningitis (markedly elevated protein, normal or low glucose, and lymphocytic pleocytosis) are not always seen in cryptococcal meningitis in the setting of HIV disease. Routine CSF studies (protein, glucose, cell count) may occasionally be entirely normal in cryptococcal meningitis, highlighting the importance of the cryptococcal antigen as a diagnostic test.[1,9] In patients who refuse LP or have other contraindications to the procedure, serum cryptococcal antigen can be useful because it is only rarely negative in cryptococcal meningitis.[7]

One challenge in interpreting CSF results from patients with HIV infection is the high prevalence of mild protein elevation (<100 mg/dL) and lymphocytic pleocytosis (<50/mm^3). More marked abnormalities in CSF protein or cell count, low glucose, or polymorphonuclear pleocytosis at any CD4 count warrants investigation for causes other than HIV itself, as does pleocytosis in patients with CD4 count of less than 50/mm^3 or whose HIV disease is well controlled on ART.[16] If the CSF profile resembles bacterial meningitis, with elevated protein, polymorphonuclear pleocytosis, and low or normal glucose, an additional diagnostic consideration, particularly in patients with CD4 counts less than 50 cells/mm^3, is CMV ventriculoencephalitis. In such patients, CT may be normal or reveal mild hydrocephalus, periventricular enhancement, or both.[17] CSF PCR for CMV nucleic acids can establish the diagnosis.

Patients whose AMS remains unexplained after blood work, CT, and CSF examination may require an electroencephalogram (EEG) to exclude nonconvulsive status epilepticus.

COMPLICATIONS AND ADMISSION CRITERIA

Except for patients with a secure diagnosis of a rapidly reversible and definitively treatable toxic-metabolic encephalopathy, such as hypoglycemia or opiate overdose, or seizure with full recovery (and negative workup), most patients with AMS and HIV disease require admission. Patients with focal CNS infection, meningitis, or PCNSL are at risk for seizures and increased ICP, although antiepileptic drugs (AEDs) are not given as routine prophylaxis without a documented seizure. Elevated ICP may develop as a consequence of focal or generalized cerebral edema, hydrocephalus, or both. Patients with meningitis may develop cranial neuropathies, and ischemic stroke may complicate syphilitic, tuberculous, or acute bacterial meningitis.

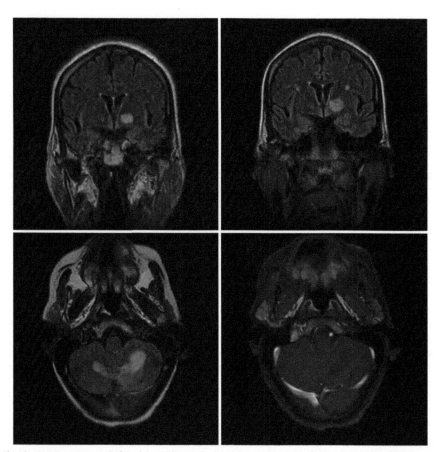

Fig. 3. Progressive multifocal leukoencephalopathy. Brain MRI from an AIDS patient who presented with mental status change and ataxia showed left basal ganglia (*top left*) and left cerebellum (*bottom left*) lesions without mass effect on FLAIR images. Repeat brain MRI 2 months later (*top right*) showed increase in the size of the basal ganglia lesion as well as interval development of a smaller lesion in the left frontal white matter. T1-weighted MRI post gadolinium demonstrated no enhancement of the left cerebellar lesion (*bottom right*) or the left frontal lobe and basal ganglia lesions (not shown). Positive CSF JC virus polymerase chain reaction confirmed the diagnosis of progressive multifocal leukoencephalopathy.

TREATMENT AND PROPHYLAXIS

Therapy may not always be started in the acute care setting for HIV-related cerebral OIs if there is significant diagnostic uncertainty and no indication of neurologic emergency (ie, no increased ICP, seizure, bacterial meningitis, or acute stroke) (**Table 5**).

Increased ICP is managed in the usual fashion, as is status epilepticus. The recurrence risk for seizures in patients with HIV disease appears to be higher than in seronegative patients[18]; hence it is reasonable to consider AED therapy for a single seizure, in the absence of an obvious reversible toxic-metabolic precipitant such as withdrawal, cocaine or methamphetamine use, hypoglycemia, hyponatremia, or hypocalcemia. That decision is particularly complicated in patients on ART, because first-line AEDs such as phenytoin and carbamazepine, as hepatic enzyme inducers, have

Table 5
Initial treatment of selected CNS infections in HIV/AIDS

Cerebral toxoplasmosis	• Pyrimethamine 200 mg PO loading dose then 50 mg (<60 kg) or 75 mg ($\geq$60 kg) PO daily plus sulfadiazine 1 g (<60 kg) or 1.5 g ($\geq$60 kg) PO every 6 h plus folinic acid 10–20 mg PO daily • Consult infectious diseases specialist for patients with antibiotic allergies or who cannot take oral medications
Cryptococcal meningitis	• Amphotericin B 0.7 mg/kg IV daily plus flucytosine 25 mg/kg/d PO every 6 h (caution if significant marrow failure) • Consult infectious disease specialist for patients with renal insufficiency, for consideration of liposomal amphotericin • Consider high-dose oral fluconazole 400–800 mg PO daily, with flucytosine 25 mg/kg/d PO every 6 h (caution if significant marrow failure) for patients who decline admission, lack intravenous access, or cannot tolerate amphotericin
PML	• None (ART in treatment-naïve patients)
Tuberculous meningitis	• Four-drug therapy; consult infectious disease specialist due to complex drug-drug interactions between many antituberculous drugs, particularly rifampin, and many ART regimens • Consider adjunctive dexamethasone (may be started after antituberculous drugs begun)
Neurosyphilis	• Penicillin G 18–24 million units per day (3–4 million units IV every 4 h or continuous infusion) *or* • Procaine penicillin 2.4 million units IM once daily plus probenecid 500 mg PO 4 times a day (if adherence with daily injections and oral probenecid can be assured)
VZV encephalitis	• Acyclovir 10–15 mg/kg IV every 8 h
CMV encephalitis	• Ganciclovir with or without foscarnet; consult infectious disease specialist
Bacterial meningitis (community-acquired)	• Consider adjunctive dexamethasone, 10–20 min before or at the same time as initial dose of antibiotics, 0.15 mg/kg every 6 h for proven or suspected pneumococcal meningitis • Cover for *Listeria monocytogenes* (ampicillin or penicillin), in addition to meningococcus and pneumococcus (ceftriaxone and vancomycin): vancomycin 30–45 mg/kg/d IV divided every 8–12 h + ceftriaxone 4 g/d IV divided every 12 h (or once daily) + ampicillin 1–2 g/day IV divided every 4 h In penicillin-allergic patients, ampicillin should be substituted with trimethoprim-sulfamethoxazole 10–20 mg/kg trimethoprim component divided every 6–12 h

Abbreviations: IM, intramuscular; IV, intravenous; PO, by mouth.
  Data from[7,8,15]

adverse drug-drug interactions with most ART regimens.[19] Failure of antiretroviral therapy has been reported in this context, highlighting the importance of prescribing with great care in patients on ART.[20]

Current general treatment guidelines recommend adjunctive dexamethasone with antimycobacterial agents for patients with tuberculous meningitis and dexamethasone before or with the first dose of antibiotics in patients with community-acquired acute bacterial meningitis.[21,22] The data regarding steroids in HIV-infected patients with these infections are scant. The Centers for Disease Control and Prevention recommend adjuvant dexamethasone or prednisone for tuberculous meningitis or CNS tuberculoma in HIV-infected patients,[7] while the Cochrane Collaboration recommends routine use of steroids in non-HIV–infected patients and notes insufficient data to advise for or against a similar approach in non-HIV–infected patients.[23] In bacterial meningitis, a recent study from Africa, in which 90% of the participants were HIV-infected and showed no survival benefit with adjunctive dexamethasone,[24] contrasts strikingly with current treatment guidelines and illustrates the need for further study on the role of adjunctive steroids in bacterial meningitis with and without HIV coinfection in high- and low-income countries.

In patients with IRIS, ART is usually continued; steroids are sometimes administered to attenuate the inflammatory response, although controlled data are lacking.

SUMMARY

Key elements of the history in HIV-infected patients with AMS include recent and nadir CD4 count, recent viral load, prior neurologic or psychiatric disorders, and detailed medication history, including antibiotic use and allergies, illicit and other nonprescribed drugs, and composition and duration of ART regimen. AMS in the first weeks to months of ART may be medication-related if efavirenz is one of the prescribed drugs, or may be due to an immune reconstitution relapse of tuberculous or cryptococcal meningitis or PML. The risk of major cerebral OIs and malignancies is highest for patients with CD4 counts less than 200 cells/mm^3. The absence of headache, fever, or meningismus should not be used to exclude these diagnoses. Noncontrast head CT is indicated in the evaluation of AMS in HIV-infected patients; contrast-enhanced CT should be considered in patients with CD4 counts less than 200 cells/mm^3 or symptoms or signs of focal cerebral dysfunction. Cerebral toxoplasmosis is a common cause of fever and focal cerebral dysfunction in patients with AIDS and ring-enhancing lesions on neuroimaging studies; *Toxoplasma* IgG serology is usually positive. AIDS patients with headache may have cryptococcal meningitis, even with normal mental status, nonfocal examination, and normal neuroimaging. Serum cryptococcal antigen can help suggest or exclude the diagnosis in patients who refuse or have other contraindications to LP. Medications should be prescribed carefully for patients on ART, because of complex drug-drug interactions, particularly for hepatic enzyme-inducing agents such as rifampin and older antiepileptic drugs.

REFERENCES

1. Mamidi A, DeSimone JA, Pomerantz RJ. Central nervous system infections in individuals with HIV-1 infection. J Neurovirol 2002;8(3):158–67.
2. Treisman GJ, Kaplin AI. Neurologic and psychiatric complications of antiretroviral agents. AIDS 2002;16(9):1201–15.
3. Sacktor N. The epidemiology of human immunodeficiency virus-associated neurological disease in the era of highly active antiretroviral therapy. J Neurovirol 2002;8(Suppl 2):115–21.
4. Riedel DJ, Pardo CA, McArthur JC, et al. Therapy insight: CNS manifestations of HIV-associated immune reconstitution inflammatory syndrome. Nat Clin Pract Neurol 2006;2(10):557–65.
5. Janssen RS, Cornblath DR, Epstein LG, et al. Human immunodeficiency virus (HIV) infection and the nervous system: report from the American Academy of Neurology AIDS Task Force. Neurology 1989;39(1):119–22.

6. Kanzer MD. Neuropathology of AIDS. Crit Rev Neurobiol 1990;5(4):313–62.
7. Centers for Disease Control and Prevention. Guidelines for prevention and treatment of opportunistic infections in HIV-infected adults and adolescents: recommendations from CDC, the National Institutes of Health, and the HIV Medicine Association of the Infectious Diseases Society of America. MMWR 2009;58(No. RR04):1–198.
8. Portegies P, Solod L, Cinque P, et al. Guidelines for the diagnosis and management of neurological complications of HIV infection. Eur J Neurol 2004;11(5): 297–304.
9. Manji H, Miller R. The neurology of HIV infection. J Neurol Neurosurg Psychiatr 2004;75(Suppl 1):i29–35.
10. Murdoch DM, Venter WDF, Van Rie A, et al. Immune reconstitution inflammatory syndrome (IRIS): review of common infectious manifestations and treatment options. AIDS Res Ther 2007;4:9.
11. Clifford DB, Yang Y, Evans S. Neurologic consequences of hepatitis C and human immunodeficiency virus coinfection. J Neurovirol 2005;11(Suppl 3):67–71.
12. Rothman RE, Keyl PM, McArthur JC, et al. A decision guideline for emergency department utilization of noncontrast head computerized tomography in HIV-infected patients. Acad Emerg Med 1999;6(10):1010–9.
13. Tso EL, Todd WC, Groleau GA, et al. Cranial computed tomography in the emergency department evaluation of HIV-infected patients with neurologic complaints. Ann Emerg Med 1993;22(7):1169–76.
14. Smith AB, Smirniotopoulos JG, Rushing EJ. From the archives of the AFIP: central nervous system infections associated with human immunodeficiency virus infection: radiologic-pathologic correlation. Radiographics 2008;28(7):2033–58.
15. Saag MS, Graybill RJ, Larsen RA, et al. Practice guidelines for the management of cryptococcal disease. Clin Infect Dis 2000;30(4):710–8.
16. Spudich SS, Nilsson AC, Lollo ND, et al. Cerebrospinal fluid HIV infection and pleocytosis: relation to systemic infection and antiretroviral treatment. BMC Infect Dis 2005;5:98.
17. Arribas JR, Storch GA, Clifford DB, et al. Cytomegalovirus encephalitis. Ann Intern Med 1996;125(7):577–87.
18. Romanelli F, Ryan M. Seizures in HIV-seropositive individuals: epidemiology and treatment. CNS Drugs 2002;12(2):91–8.
19. Liedtke MD, Lockhart SM, Rathbun RC. Anticonvulsant and antiretroviral interactions. Ann Pharmcother 2004;38(3):482–9.
20. McNichol IR, editor. HIVInSite database of antiretroviral drug interactions. Available at: http://hivinsite.ucsf.edu/arvdb?page=ar-0002. Accessed August 17, 2009.
21. Centers for Disease Control and Prevention. Treatment of tuberculosis: American Thoracic Society, CDC, and Infectious Diseases Society of America. MMWR 2003;52(RR11):1–77.
22. Tunkel AR, Hartman BJ, Kaplan SL, et al. Practice guidelines for the management of bacterial meningitis. Clin Infect Dis 2004;39(9):1267–84.
23. Prasad K, Singh SB. Corticosteroids for managing tuberculous meningitis. Cochrane Database Syst Rev 2008;(1):CD002244. DOI:10.1002/14651858:CD002244.pub3.
24. Scarborough M, Gordon SB, Whitty CJM, et al. Corticosteroids for bacterial meningitis in adults in Sub-Saharan Africa. N Engl J Med 2007;357(24):2441–50.

Emergency Department Management of Hematologic and Oncologic Complications in the Patient Infected with HIV

Sara B. Scott, MD

KEYWORDS

- HIV • AIDS • Thrombocytopenia • Anemia
- Malignancy • Thrombosis

HEMATOLOGIC CONSIDERATIONS IN THE PATIENT INFECTED WITH HUMAN IMMUNODEFICIENCY VIRUS

Blood dyscrasias are common in the setting of human immunodeficiency virus (HIV) infection. Anemia, neutropenia, and thrombocytopenia are some of the most frequent blood abnormalities found in patients with HIV infection presenting to the emergency department (ED). In addition, patients with HIV suffer from more complex hematologic diagnoses with greater frequency than the general population, including immune thrombocytopenic purpura (ITP), thrombotic thrombocytopenic purpura (TTP), and venous thromboses.

Anemia

Anemia is the most common cytopenia in patients with HIV, although estimates of prevalence vary widely from 1.3% to 95%. The exact prevalence of anemia in this patient population is difficult to determine because of the group's diversity in age, disease severity, and comorbidities. Despite the heterogeneity of this patient population, anemia is a consistent, independent risk factor for mortality in patients with HIV. Survival is proportional to the severity of anemia, with the most severely anemic patients portending the greatest risk of death.[1]

Although anemia indicates a poorer prognosis in individuals infected with HIV, recovery from anemia has been found to improve survival.[1] Accordingly, the

Department of Emergency Medicine, University of Maryland School of Medicine, 22 South Greene Street, Baltimore, MD 21201, USA
E-mail address: sscot005@umaryland.edu

Emerg Med Clin N Am 28 (2010) 325–333
doi:10.1016/j.emc.2010.01.007   emed.theclinics.com
0733-8627/10/$ – see front matter © 2010 Published by Elsevier Inc.

identification of anemia in patients with HIV infection is essential, so that reversible causes can be diagnosed and corrected. Although a full evaluation for causes of anemia is outside the scope of practice of the emergency physician, 2 simple, readily available laboratory studies (reticulocyte count and mean corpuscular volume [MCV]) can help to narrow down the causes of the anemia and direct a pathway for a more extensive work-up by the patient's primary care provider or HIV specialist.

A reticulocyte count less than 2% indicates that the bone marrow is not increasing red cell production in response to a patient's anemia and can be categorized as hypoproliferative anemia. Further differentiation of hypoproliferative anemia can be derived by examining the MCV of the patient's red blood cells as shown in **Table 1**.

A reticulocyte count greater than 2% indicates that the bone marrow is responding to the patient's anemia by generating more red blood cell precursors. Causes of anemia in this group of patients include[2]

- Autoimmune hemolysis
- Oxidant drugs in the setting of glucose-6-phosphate dehydrogenase deficiency
- Disseminated intravascular coagulation
- TTP
- Response to acute blood loss
- Response to iron, folate, or vitamin B_{12} therapy.

Nearly half of all cases of anemia are caused by medications, and common offenders include zidovudine [formerly AZT (Retrovir)], trimethoprim-sulfamethoxazole (Bactrim, Septra, Sulfatrim), and ganciclovir (Cytovene, Cymevene).[3] A more extensive list of medications that can cause anemia in this patient population is listed in **Table 2**.

Although cessation of the offending drug may improve anemia, these agents should not be stopped abruptly, as this may result in serious infectious complications and resistance to future treatment.[2] Any substitutions or alterations in the medication regimen should be discussed with the patient's primary care provider or HIV specialist.

Symptomatic or severe anemia requires immediate intervention. Although an association between transfusions and mortality in individuals with HIV infection has been found in some studies,[4] the transfusion criteria for patients with HIV does not differ from the general population. Persistent symptoms, cardiac compromise, respiratory distress, and/or hemoglobin <8 g/dL are fairly standard indications for transfusion of packed red blood cells in this patient population.[2] Obtaining iron studies, reticulocyte count, and bilirubin levels, before the transfusion of blood products may expedite the inpatient work-up.

Table 1 Differential diagnosis of hypoproliferative anemia in the patient infected with HIV	
Low MCV (<80 fL)	• Iron deficiency • Thalassemia
Normal MCV (80–100 fL)	• Anemia of chronic disease • Antiviral drugs • Bone marrow tumor • Bone marrow infection
High MCV (>100 fL)	• Medications • Cancer chemotherapy • Folate deficiency

Data from Claster S. Biology of anemia, differential diagnosis and treatment options in human immunodeficiency virus infection. J Infect Dis 2002;185(Suppl 2):S105–9.

Table 2 Medications with the potential to cause anemia in HIV-infected patients	
Antiretrovirals agents	• Zidovudine • Lamivudine (Epivir, 3TC) • Didanosine (ddl, Videx) • Stavudine (Zerit)
Prophylactic anti-infective agents	• Sulfonamides • Pyrimethamine (Daraprim) • Pentamidine (Pentam)
Antiviral agents	• Ganciclovir • Foscarnet (Foscavir) • Cidofovir (Vistide) • Ribavirin (Copegus, Rebetol, Ribasphere)
Antifungal agents	• Flucytosine (Ancobon) • Amphotericin B (Fungilin, Fungizone, Abelcet, AmBisome, Fungisome, Amphocil, Amphotec)

Data from Levine AM. Hematologic manifestations of AIDS. In: Hoffman R, Benz EJ, Shattil SJ, et al, editors. Hematology: basic principles and practice. 5th edition. Philadelphia: Churchill Livingstone Elsevier; 2009.

Neutropenia

Like anemia, neutropenia is also common in individuals with HIV. The neutropenia is usually mild and of little clinical significance.[3] The same myelosuppressive drugs that cause anemia (zidovudine, trimethoprim-sulfamethoxazole, ganciclovir) are often responsible for a decreased neutrophil count. In addition, infiltration of the bone marrow by mycobacteria or neoplastic cells can lead to a diminished number of circulating neutrophils.[5] When the neutropenia is clinically significant, it is often in association with antineoplastic agents used to treat HIV-associated malignancies.[3] Granulocyte colony-stimulating factor is sometimes used to treat these individuals, but is generally not a drug initiated in the ED.

Although the neutropenia in individuals infected with HIV is usually mild and of little clinical significance, care should be exercised when evaluating patients with HIV with more severe neutropenia, as they are at increased risk for serious bacterial infections. In patients with an absolute neutrophil count (ANC) less than 1000 cells/mm^3 there is a 2-fold increase in bacterial infection. This increases to nearly 8-fold when the ANC falls to less than 500 cells/mm^3.[6] The lower the CD4 count in patients with HIV with neutropenia, the higher the risk of bacterial infection.[6] Certainly patients with HIV infection presenting to the ED with an ANC less than 1000 cells/mm^3 and fever should be extensively evaluated for infection, including cultures, and provided with empiric antibiotics until culture results have returned.

Thrombocytopenia

Thrombocytopenia is also a common abnormality associated with HIV infection. Fortunately, it is rarely associated with bleeding.[3] Causes of thrombocytopenia in individuals infected with HIV include

- TTP
- ITP
- Hemolytic uremic syndrome (HUS)

- Opportunistic infection
- Malignancy
- Medications
- Concomitant liver disease
- Alcohol abuse
- Splenomegaly.

The most common cause of thrombocytopenia in patients with HIV is ITP.[6]

ITP

ITP is a result of increased destruction of platelets by the spleen. In patients with HIV, this is exacerbated by diminished production of platelets and decreased platelet survival.[6] Despite being the most frequent cause of thrombocytopenia in patients with HIV, ITP is a diagnosis of exclusion, requiring a thorough diagnostic evaluation for other causes of thrombocytopenia before its diagnosis.

ITP may resolve spontaneously and typically requires no treatment. However, treatment is recommended in patients with active bleeding, platelet count less than 30,000/μL or less than 50,000/μL with underlying coagulopathy (eg, hemophilia), or in patients undergoing invasive procedures.[6] Transfusion of platelets will not alter the underlying autoimmune destruction of platelets and will only serve as an interim treatment. Long-term therapy is with antiretroviral therapy (ART), interferon-alpha, high-dose intravenous gamma globulin (IVIG), anti-Rh immunoglobulin, or even splenectomy.[6] Although corticosteroids are the mainstay of therapy for most patients with ITP, they are not currently recommended for HIV-related ITP because of their immunosuppressive effects and the risk for the development of fulminant Kaposi sarcoma (KS).[6]

TTP

Another potential cause of thrombocytopenia in individuals infected with HIV is TTP. TTP is more common in individuals infected with HIV than in the general population.[3] It is characterized by a thrombotic microangiopathy that results in widespread thromboses forming in small blood vessels. This subsequently leads to thrombocytopenia via the consumption of platelets. The 5 cardinal symptoms of TTP are thrombocytopenia, fever, hemolytic anemia, renal dysfunction, and neurologic abnormalities such as headache, seizure, or coma. Platelet transfusion for the treatment of thrombocytopenia associated with TTP is contraindicated, as it can worsen intravascular clotting. For this reason, it is absolutely essential that the emergency physician recognize the cause of thrombocytopenia as TTP and refrain from administering platelets to these patients. Instead, treatment of TTP is accomplished by plasmapheresis or plasma exchange, which should be initiated as soon as possible to minimize damage to the kidneys and brain.[7]

Thrombosis

In addition to coagulation abnormalities secondary to platelet pathology, HIV infection has also been associated with coagulation abnormalities leading to increased incidence of venous thromboembolism. In fact, 1 recent study found that individuals with HIV infection were 4 times more likely to develop deep vein thrombosis (DVT) than age-matched counterparts in the general population.[8] Consequently, HIV infection is an important risk factor that the emergency physician needs to take into consideration when entertaining the diagnosis of DVT or pulmonary embolism. Further risk stratification includes the patient's CD4 count and any current infection, as the mean CD4 count of patients with HIV with venous thromboembolism is often less than 200 cells/mm^3 and ongoing infection is associated with an increased risk.[8]

Treatment of thromboembolic disease in the patient with HIV is the same as for the general population, but maintenance of a therapeutic international normalized ratio can be more difficult in this patient population because of the interaction of warfarin (Coumadin) with many of the protease inhibitors.

ONCOLOGIC CONSIDERATIONS IN THE HIV-INFECTED PATIENT

The prevalence of a multitude of cancers is increased in the HIV population. These include AIDS-defining conditions, such as KS, invasive cervical carcinoma, and non-Hodgkin lymphoma (NHL) as well as other malignancies like Hodgkin lymphoma, anal cancer, lung cancer, multiple myeloma, angiosarcoma, and seminoma.[9] ED management of most of these conditions will not be altered for the patient infected with HIV, compared with the general population. However, there are a couple of key concepts for the emergency physician to understand, particularly in the management and evaluation of KS, NHL (more specifically primary central nervous system lymphoma), and the anogenital carcinomas. These topics are discussed in this section in more depth.

KS

KS, once affecting up to 33% of patients with AIDS, now affects less than 1% of patients with AIDS in the United States.[10] However, even with this decline in prevalence since the advent of ART, KS is still the most common malignancy in patients with AIDS in the United States[10] and is considered an AIDS-defining clinical condition. Although the prevalence of KS is highest in homosexual men, the disease has been found to affect other groups as well.[11]

KS is a virus-related tumor associated with human herpesvirus 8 (HHV8). KS may present with cutaneous findings including palpable, nontender nodules, or nonpalpable macules resembling ecchymosis. In light-skinned individuals lesions may be purplish-blue, whereas in dark-skinned individuals they may appear brownish-black. Skin lesions are most common on the face, lower extremities, and genitalia and may be associated with extensive lymphedema. Oral lesions occur in up to one-third of affected individuals.[12] KS should be included in the differential diagnosis of any patient infected with HIV presenting with new rash, oral lesions, or lymphedema. Skin biopsy can confirm the diagnosis.

KS can involve nearly every part of the body, but 3 common areas that the emergency physician should investigate closely include the gastrointestinal (GI) system, pulmonary system, and larynx. In the latter, airway obstruction can occur when KS infiltrates the larynx.[13] Vigilance should be used when examining any patient with KS with complaints of sore throat, cough, dysphagia, hoarseness, hemoptysis, or other airway-related complaints.[13] Airway management in the emergent situation is the same as for any patient with airway obstruction. In the nonemergent situation, consultation with otolaryngology may aid in defining the location and extent of obstruction to further guide management.

Infiltration of the GI system by KS may present as nausea, anorexia, abdominal pain, and weight loss. Less frequently, KS may clinically manifest as perforation, bleeding, or obstruction.[11,12] GI KS may occur in the absence of cutaneous disease and is present in nearly 40% of patients at the time of initial diagnosis.[11,12] Accordingly, KS should be considered in the differential diagnosis of patients with HIV infection presenting with the aforementioned GI symptoms. Diagnosis is confirmed by endoscopy.

The pulmonary system can also be affected by KS, causing cough, dyspnea, fever, and/or hemoptysis. Chest radiographs in these patients may reveal bronchial wall thickening, nodules, Kerly B lines, and/or pleural effusions.[14] Like GI infiltration, pulmonary infiltration by KS may occur in the absence of cutaneous disease and consideration should be given to KS in the differential diagnosis of patients with HIV presenting with respiratory symptoms. Diagnosis is made by bronchoscopy.

The identification of patients with KS is crucial as administration of corticosteroids in these patients has been associated with exacerbation of the disease process. Although a recent study did not find any increase in the incidence of KS in patients treated with corticosteroids for *Pneumocystis jiroveci* pneumonia,[15] corticosteroid use has been attributed to 1 KS-related death in a patient with AIDS being treated for immune reconstitution syndrome.[16] Because of the controversial and evolving nature of this issue, consultation with an infectious disease specialist is recommended before initiating corticosteroids in patients with HIV infection with KS.

NHL

NHL is a term that encompasses all malignancies of the lymphoid system except for Hodgkin lymphoma. Like KS, NHL is more prevalent in individuals infected with HIV than in individuals without HIV with an incidence of 60 times that of the general population.[11] AIDS-related NHLs are usually aggressive high-grade lymphomas of B cell origin.[17] Diffuse large B cell lymphoma (DLBCL) and Burkitt lymphoma are the most common AIDS-related lymphomas (ARL), representing approximately 90% of all ARLs.[12]

Patients with systemic NHL typically present with lymphadenopathy. A high level of suspicion should be maintained for NHL in patients infected with HIV presenting with lymphadenopathy. Associated B-symptoms (fever, night sweats, and weight loss) are more common in patients with ARL than in NHL patients without HIV,[3,12] and should be included in the review of systems for patients with HIV with lymphadenopathy. Extranodal involvement is also more common in individuals infected with HIV with NHL than in individuals without HIV with NHL. The bone marrow, meninges, and GI tract are the most frequently involved extranodal sites.[11]

In contrast with patients affected by systemic NHL, patients with primary central nervous system lymphoma (PCNSL) have disease confined to the central nervous system. PCNSL is most often DLBCL histology and carries a poor prognosis with median survival of 1 to 2.5 months with supportive care alone.[18] PCNSL is the most common brain malignancy in patients infected with HIV[19] and the second most common intracranial mass lesion in AIDS patients.[18] Presenting symptoms for PCNSL include altered mental status, motor deficits, cranial nerve palsies, headache, and seizures.[18] Thus, a high index of suspicion should be maintained for patients infected with HIV presenting with any neurologic complaints, particularly if the CD4 count is known to be less than 200 cells/mm^3. ED work-up should include a head computed tomography (CT) scan with and without contrast. PCNSL may be isodense, hypodense, or hyperdense on noncontrast CT, however, with contrast administration PCNSL lesions nearly always enhance.[18] Unfortunately, the clinical presentation and appearance on CT of PCNSL can make it difficult to differentiate from toxoplasmosis. Some general guidelines focusing on the radiologic characteristics of the lesions (**Table 3**) can aid in differentiating between PCNSL and toxoplasmosis.[20]

ED work-up should also consist of a lumbar puncture if there is no evidence of increased intracranial pressure on CT. Laboratory analysis for serologic and cerebrospinal fluid (CSF) toxoplasmosis as well as for CSF Epstein-Barr virus (EBV) may help to further distinguish PCNSL from toxoplasmosis.[17] EBV DNA is found in all cases of PCNSL.[11] Toxoplasma seronegativity coupled with the presence of EBV detected by polymerase chain reaction performed on CSF is highly suggestive of PCNSL. Although

Table 3				
Radiologic characteristics that aid in the differentiation of PCNSL and toxoplasmosis				
	Lesion Location	**Number of Lesions**	**Size of Lesions**	**Contrast Enhancement of Lesion**
PCNSL	Variable	Solitary or multiple	2–6 cm	Diffuse, homogeneous
Toxoplasmosis	Basal ganglia and gray-white junctions	Multiple	<2 cm	Ring-enhancing

Data from Taiwo BO. AIDS-related primary CNS lymphoma: a brief review. AIDS Read 2000; 10(80):486–91.

ultimately this may not be a diagnosis that is made in the ED, a thorough initial evaluation can certainly expedite the inpatient work-up and hasten appropriate treatment.

Anogenital Neoplasias

Individuals infected with HIV are also at increased risk for cervical and anal cancer.[21] The Centers for Disease Control includes invasive cervical cancer as an AIDS-defining illness. Compared with the general population, women with HIV infection more often have multifocal cervical cancer, which may involve the vagina and vulva.[11] Invasive cervical cancer and invasive squamous cell carcinoma of the anus are associated with human papillomavirus (HPV), the virus responsible for genital and anal warts. Thus, any individual infected with HIV with lesions of the anogenital system or evidence of HPV infection presenting to the ED should be urgently referred for follow-up Pap smear and anoscopy because of their increased risk of invasive malignant lesions.

SUMMARY

Although many of the hematologic and oncologic diseases affecting people with HIV also affect the general population, they seem to be more prevalent in those with HIV. This may be a direct result of HIV infection, medication side effects, or opportunistic infections. Regardless of the cause, the diagnosis of a cytopenia or a malignancy in this patient population often portends greater mortality than in the general population. Although ED management of many of the hematologic and oncologic complications of HIV do not differ drastically from the management of these conditions in the general population, the recognition of these conditions in patients infected with HIV is of paramount importance for identifying patients at high risk of morbidity and mortality. The early diagnosis of these disease processes and the establishment of appropriate care and follow-up are essential to optimize patient outcomes.

REFERENCES

1. Belpario PS, Rhew DC. Prevalence and outcomes of anemia in individuals with human immunodeficiency virus: a systematic review of the literature. Am J Med 2004;116(7A):27S–43S.
2. Claster S. Biology of anemia, differential diagnosis and treatment options in human immunodeficiency virus infection. J Infect Dis 2002;185(Suppl 2):S105–9.
3. Sloand E. Hematologic complications of HIV infection. AIDS Rev 2005;7:187–96.
4. Buskin SE, Sullivan PS. Anemia and its treatment and outcomes in persons infected with human immunodeficiency virus. Transfusion 2004;44(6):826–32.

5. Kuritzkes DR. Neutropenia, neutrophil dysfunction, and bacterial infection in patients with human immunodeficiency virus disease: the role of granulocyte colony-stimulating factor. Clin Infect Dis 2000;30:256–60.

6. Levine AM. Hematologic manifestations of AIDS. In: Hoffman R, Benz EJ, Shattil SJ, et al, editors. Hematology: basic principles and practice. 5th edition. Philadelphia: Churchill Livingstone Elsevier; 2009. p. 2321–38. Available at: https://remote.mdmercy. com/book/player/,DanaInfo=www.mdconsult.com+book.do?method=display&type= bookPage&decorator=header&eid=4-u1.0-B978-0-443-06715-0..50160-6& uniq=189663205&isbn=978-0-443-06715-0&sid=969407606#lpState=open&lpTab= contentsTab&content=4-u1.0-B978-0-443-06715-0..50160-6-cesec1%3Bfrom%3Dcontent% 3Bisbn%3D978-0-443-06715-0%3Btype%3DbookPage. Accessed January 15, 2010.

7. Eaton ME. Selected rare, noninfectious syndromes associated with HIV infection. Top HIV Med 2005;13(2):75–8.

8. Crum-Cianflone NF, Weekes J, Bavaro M. Thromboses among HIV-infected patients during the highly active antiretroviral therapy era. AIDS Patient Care STDS 2008;22(10):771–8.

9. Goedert JJ, Cote TR, Virgo P, et al. Spectrum of AIDS-associated malignant disorders. Lancet 1998;351:1833–9.

10. Mitchell R.N. Schoen FJ. Blood vessels In: Kumar V, Abbas AK, Fausto N, et al, editors. Robbins and Cotran pathologic basis of disease, professional edition. 8th edition. edition. Philadelphia: Saunders Elsevier; 2010. p. 487–527. Available at: https://remote.mdmercy.com/das/book/body/189663205-23/969412127/2060/, DanaInfo=www.mdconsult.com+94.html#4-u1.0-B978-1-4377-0792-2..50016-X_967. Accessed January 15, 2010.

11. Mitsuyasu R. Oncological complications of human immunodeficiency virus disease and hematologic consequences of their treatment. Clin Infect Dis 1999;29:35–43.

12. Cheung MC, Pantanowitz L, Dezube BJ. AIDS-related malignancies: emerging challenges in the era of highly active antiretroviral therapy. Oncologist 2005;10:412–26.

13. Miner JE, Egan TD. An AIDS-associated cause of the difficult airway: supraglottic Kaposi's sarcoma. Anesth Analg 2000;90:1223–6.

14. Huang L, Schnapp LM, Gruden JF, et al. Presentation of AIDS-related pulmonary Kaposi's sarcoma diagnosed by bronchoscopy. Am J Respir Crit Care Med 1996; 153(4):1385–90.

15. Gallant JE, Chaisson RE, Moore RD. The effect of adjunctive corticosteroids for the treatment of *Pneumocystis carinii* pneumonia on mortality and subsequent complications. Chest 1998;114(5):1258–63.

16. Davis JL, Shum AK, Huang L. A 36-year-old man with AIDS and relapsing, nonproductive cough. Chest 2007;131(6):1929–31.

17. Scadden DT. AIDS-related lymphomas. In: Hoffman R, Benz EJ, Shattil SJ, et al, editors. Hematology: basic principles and practice. 5th edition. Philadelphia: Churchill Livingstone Elsevier; 2009. p. 1377–85. https://remote.mdmercy.com/ book/player/,DanaInfo=www.mdconsult.com+book.do?method=display&type= bookPage&decorator=header&eid=4-u1.0-B978-0-443-06715-0..50160-6&uniq= 189663205&isbn=978-0-443-06715-0&sid=969413450#lpState=open& lpTab=contentsTab&content=4-u1.0-B978-0-443-06715-0..50088-1-cesec1%3Bfrom% 3Dindex%3Btype%3DbookPage%3Bisbn%3D978-0-443-06715-0.   Accessed January 15, 2010.

18. Kasamon YL, Ambinder RF. AIDS-related primary central nervous system lymphoma. Hematol Oncol Clin North Am 2005;19:665–87.

19. Fine HA, Mayer RJ. Primary central nervous system lymphoma. Ann Intern Med 1993;119:1093–104.
20. Taiwo BO. AIDS-related primary CNS lymphoma: a brief review. AIDS Read 2000; 10(80):486–91.
21. Spano JP, Costagliola D, Katlama C, et al. AIDS-related malignancies: state of the art and therapeutic challenges. J Clin Oncol 2008;26(29):4834–42.

Orthopedic Illnesses in Patients with HIV

Sukhjit S. Takhar, MD[a,b,*], Gregory W. Hendey, MD[a]

KEYWORDS

• HIV infection • Musculoskeletal disorder • Orthopedic illnesses

HIV infection and the medications used to treat it can cause a wide range of musculoskeletal problems.[1] Patients infected with HIV are susceptible to most of the same types of fractures, dislocations, and other musculoskeletal disorders as patients without HIV. However, there are several musculoskeletal conditions that are specific or unique to the patient infected with HIV.

The advent of antiretroviral therapy (ART) has changed the course of the disease. AIDS was transformed from an invariably fatal condition to a chronic manageable disease in developed countries.[2,3] This disease shift was accompanied by a corresponding change in the types of musculoskeletal complications that patients infected with HIV may experience. For example, there has been a decrease in opportunistic infections of the bone, and an increase in osteopenia and osteonecrosis.[4,5]

HIV, the immune response, and medications can be directly toxic to the bones, joints, and muscles. The cellular immune system is compromised and unusual organisms and malignancies can affect the host. Infections tend to present at a more advanced stage because of the underlying immune status of the patients. Certain rheumatologic conditions such as reactive arthritis (formerly Reiter syndrome) also seem to be more common in this patient population. The specific musculoskeletal conditions affecting the patient infected with HIV may be divided into 4 categories: disseminated diseases, bone disorders, joint disease, and myopathies.

DISSEMINATED DISEASES
Neoplastic

Immunosuppression predisposes patients to malignancy. Kaposi sarcoma (KS) and high-grade non-Hodgkin lymphoma (NHL) are prototypical AIDS-defining malignant diseases. A conservative estimate suggested that AIDS increases the risk of KS by

[a] UCSF-Fresno Emergency Medicine Residency Program, UCSF, 155 North Fresno Street, Fresno, CA 93701-2302, USA
[b] Division of Infectious Disease, UCSF-Fresno, Fresno, CA, USA
* Corresponding author. UCSF-Fresno Emergency Medicine Residency Program, UCSF, 155 North Fresno Street, Fresno, CA 93701-2302.
E-mail address: stakhar@fresno.ucsf.edu

Emerg Med Clin N Am 28 (2010) 335–342
doi:10.1016/j.emc.2010.01.009
0733-8627/10/$ – see front matter © 2010 Elsevier Inc. All rights reserved.

at least 310 times and NHL by more than 110-fold.[6] KS is a vascular neoplastic disease that primarily affects the skin, causing cutaneous violaceous nodules or plaques. It can involve a variety of sites including the lymph nodes, lungs, liver, and spleen. Epidemic KS is the most common AIDS-associated cancer in the United States.[6,7] There are rare reports of KS involvement of bone.[8] Generally, osseous KS is usually believed to be the result of contiguous invasion from nearby tissues.[9] KS lesions are not well visualized on plain radiographs. Other modalities such as computed tomography (CT) scan, magnetic resonance imaging (MRI), and nuclear studies are more helpful. The diagnosis should be confirmed with a biopsy of the lesion.

NHL in patients with AIDS tends to be of the aggressive B-cell type that is associated with pronounced immunosuppression. The bone marrow is involved in up 30% of cases.[10] Symptoms are variable and nonspecific. However, lymphoma presentation is often late, and patients present commonly with fever, night sweats, and weight loss. Treatment of neoplastic diseases in HIV patients involves a team approach with an HIV specialist and an oncologist experienced in treating patients with AIDS. Treatment includes ART as well as cytotoxic drugs in NHL and widespread KS.

Infectious

Mycobacteria

Patients infected with HIV are at much higher risk for primary or reactivation of *Mycobacterium tuberculosis* (TB). The global epidemic of HIV resulted in large increases in tuberculosis (TB) rates and TB is the leading cause of death in persons infected with HIV worldwide.[11] HIV infection is also the highest risk factor for progression from latent TB to active disease.[12] TB primarily affects the pulmonary system, but in patients infected with HIV extrapulmonary manifestations are common, and may be concurrent with pulmonary TB.[11,13,14] Tuberculosis has many musculoskeletal manifestations including spondylitis, septic arthritis, osteomyelitis, and bursitis.[13] Extrapulmonary tuberculosis is believed to be the result of hematogenous dissemination and seeding of remote sites by the mycobacterium. A common site for musculoskeletal tuberculosis is the lower thoracic or the upper lumbar segments of the vertebral column (Pott disease). A case series from Zambia revealed that two-thirds of patients with musculoskeletal TB had spinal involvement (**Table 1**).[15]

Untreated tuberculous spondylitis results in progressive inflammation and necrosis of the bone, causing vertebral collapse. Ten percent of these patients can develop neurologic complications.[1] Large paraspinal abscesses are also characteristic of TB. There can also be soft tissue extension leading to psoas muscle involvement.[1]

Table 1
Musculoskeletal manifestations of tuberculosis in patients infected with HIV in Zambia (N=188)

Location	n (%)
Spinal disease	124 (66)
Hip disease	35 (18)
Knee	19 (10)
Other joints	9 (6)
Other bone	2 (1)

Data from Jellis JE. Orthopaedic surgery and HIV disease in Africa. Int Orthop 1996;20(4):253–6.

MRI of the spine is the initial diagnostic modality of choice, as plain film findings may be absent. A bone biopsy will confirm the diagnosis.

Tuberculosis can also seed a joint space causing septic arthritis. It preferentially affects the large weight-bearing joints such as the hip and knee (see **Table 1**). In these cases the patients often have concurrent osteomyelitis and soft tissue involvement.[13] Clinical findings are nonspecific and a bone biopsy with a positive tuberculin skin test is needed to make the diagnosis.

Atypical mycobacterial infections are a manifestation of advanced AIDS. They are not as pathogenic and the risk of systemic dissemination increases when the CD4 count decreases to less than 100 cells/mm^3.[16] There are many reports of musculo-skeletal infections from atypical mycobactera in the literature. These infections occur late in the disease process and are often associated with other opportunistic infections. Atypical mycobacterial infections generally spread hematogenously and often involve several joints or bony sites. Even though *Mycobacterium avium complex* is the most common atypical mycobacterial infection in patients with HIV, *Mycobacterium kansasii and Mycobacterium haemophilum* have more of a predilection for the musculoskeletal system. Cutaneous lesions such as nodules and ulcers are often present and may be a clue to the diagnosis.[13,17]

Bartonella

Bacillary angiomatosis (BA) is a disseminated infection that is caused by *Bartonella henselae* and *Bartonella quintana*. The organism involved is a rickettsia-like organism. In the immunocompetent host, *Bartonella henselae* cause a local self-limited lymphadenitis. It is associated with cutaneous and visceral involvement in those with advanced AIDS. The vascular proliferative lesions in the skin are difficult to distinguish clinically from KS.[18] Involvement of the lymph nodes, central nervous system (CNS), liver, and osteomyelitis, especially in the long bones [1,13] occur in advanced AIDS. In fact, osteomyelitis may differentiate BA from KS as bony involvement is an unusual manifestation of KS. Again, the diagnosis is made with a bone biopsy, and antibiotic therapy can be curative. Untreated disease can be fatal.

BONE DISORDERS
Osteopenia and Osteoporosis

Normal bone undergoes continuous remodeling, with matched bony resorption and new bone formation. Multiple studies have suggested patients infected with HIV have lower bone mineral density (BMD) than age-matched controls.[4,19,20] The causes are many, and include the disease itself as well as medications.

BMD can be measured using dual x-ray absorptiometry (DXA), single x-ray absorptiometry (SXA), and quantitative CT scan. Osteoporosis is defined by a bone density that is greater than 2.5 standard deviations (SD) from normal, which is based on a young control group. Osteopenia is defined as a BMD that is 1 to 2.5 SD less than normal. The reduction in the strength of the bone leads to an increased risk of fractures.[20] In 1 recent series, fractures of the spine, hip, and wrist were significantly more common in patients infected with HIV than in controls with no HIV infection (**Table 2**). The pathogenesis of osteoporosis is complicated and multifactorial.

ART, especially protease inhibitors, have been linked to the development of osteopenia and osteoporosis.[4,20] In addition, HIV is now believed to be an independent risk factor for reduced BMD. Currently, bone densitometry is recommended in women infected with HIV aged 65 years or older and in younger women with additional risk factors for premature bone loss.[21] Osteoporosis is often under diagnosed in men and HIV is a significant risk factor.[22]

Table 2 Increased incidence of fractures in patients infected with HIV		
	Infected with HIV	**Not Infected with HIV**
Total fractures	2.87/100 persons	1.77/100 persons
Vertebral	1.01/100 persons	0.47/100 persons
Hip	0.72/100 persons	0.51/100 persons
Wrist	1.38/100 persons	0.90/100 persons

Data from Triant VA, Brown TT, Lee H, et al. Fracture prevalence among human immunodeficiency virus (HIV)-infected versus non-HIV infected patients in a large U.S. healthcare system. J Clin Endocrinol Metab 2008;93(9):3499–504.

Osteonecrosis

Osteonecrosis, previously known as avascular necrosis, refers to bone infarction at the epiphyseal regions of a bone near a joint. The incidence of osteonecrosis is up to 45 times greater in patients infected with HIV.[23] Traditional predisposing factors include hypertriglyceridemia, corticosteroid use, and ethanol abuse. ART, especially protease inhibitors, have also been implicated.[1,4,23] Osteonecrosis occurs most often in the femoral head, but may occur in other locations. Although the risk factors have not been completely elucidated, a lower CD4 count and a history of corticosteroid use are associated with its development.

Unfortunately, benign musculoskeletal complaints are common in HIV patients, but the emergency physician must maintain a high index of suspension in patients presenting with severe, persistent, or unusual pain. Routine radiographic screening in asymptomatic patients is not recommended.[21] MRI of the hip is recommended in patients with persistent pain and in those who have abnormal plain radiographs. Orthopedic referral is needed in those patients with a suspicion of osteonecrosis.[21,23]

Osteomyelitis

Osteomyelitis, or infection of the bone, is a heterogeneous disease process and may result from hematogenous spread of a remote infection, local spread of a contiguous focus of infection, or direct inoculation.[24] The disease may be divided into acute and chronic forms. Excluding BA, osteomyelitis in the patient infected with HIV is similar to that in patients without HIV, and is a relatively uncommon complication. However, when osteomyelitis occurs, many organisms have been reported in the patient infected with HIV, including Salmonella, Cryptococcus, Nocardia, and Candida albicans.[25] TB osteomyelitis is extremely common in endemic areas, especially when the lesion involves the vertebral column.[13] In most cases, patients are afebrile and present with back pain.

Conventional radiographs should be the first step in imaging patients with suspected osteomyelitis. When positive, they are helpful; however, normal plain films are unable to exclude the diagnosis of osteomyelitis. A 30% to 50% reduction in bone density must occur and it can take 3 weeks for a lesion to become visible on plain films. MRI and nuclear imaging are much more sensitive and specific. MRI has become the imaging modality of choice in evaluating osteomyelitis, especially that of the vertebral column. Sensitivity is reported to be between 82% and 100% with a specificity of 75% to 96%.[25] The diagnosis is made definitively by a bone biopsy and culture. Blood cultures may be positive in bacterial osteomyelitis in cases resulting from hematogenous spread. Treatment involves long-term antimicrobial therapy and sometimes surgical debridement.[24]

JOINT DISEASE
Septic Arthritis

Septic arthritis is relatively uncommon in patients infected with HIV. Risk factors include intravenous drug use or hemophilia.[5,13,26] Infection of the joint can occur by the same mechanisms as osteomyelitis. The most common organism is *Staphylococcus aureus* regardless of HIV status. Tuberculosis is a common cause of septic arthritis in developing countries.[27] Although still rare, the risk for atypical infections, such as *Sporotrichosis schenkii* and *Candida albicans*, increases in advanced HIV.[13] Gram-negative bacilli such as *Pseudomonas aeruginosa* are found in increased incidence in patients who use intravenous drugs.

Disseminated gonococcal infection causes septic arthritis in sexually active adults. Polyarticular disease from gonococcus is more common in patients infected with HIV. The large weight-bearing joints are most often affected. Arthrocentesis and synovial fluid analysis is the mainstay of diagnosis. Patients with CD4 counts that are less than 200 cells/mm^3 may also have a lower joint fluid white blood cell count, making the diagnosis even more challenging.[26] Isolating the organism is difficult especially in atypical infections. Occasionally synovial biopsies are needed as well as special stains. Empiric treatment should be directed at methicillin-resistant *Staphylococcus aureus* (MRSA) as this is emerging as the most common cause of bacterial septic arthritis.[26,28]

Spondyloarthritis

Patients infected with HIV have a higher incidence of spondyloarthropathy than the general population. These include HLA-B27 associated reactive arthritis and psoriatic arthritis. Reactive arthritis is 100 to 200 times more common in the patient infected with HIV compared with a non-infected host.[29] However, some believe that the association of reactive arthritis with HIV is related to sexual activity and generalized immune suppression rather than the virus itself.[30] Reactive arthritis is associated with genitourinary and gastrointestinal infections like *Chlamydia trachomatis*, *Campylobacter jejuni*, and *Shigella flexneri*. Classically reactive arthritis presents with the triad of arthritis, urethritis, and conjunctivitis. Patients infected with HIV suffer a more severe and debilitating course of this disease and the classic triad is often absent.[1]

Psoriatic arthritis is up to 40 times more common in the host infected with HIV.[29] Patients may have typical changes in the skin (scaled maculopapules) of the elbows, scalp, trunk, and knees. Psoriatic arthritis is more common in those with advanced HIV disease and the skin findings are more extensive than in patients with no HIV infection.[31] Psoriatic arthritis often involves the surrounding tendons and fascia (enthesopathy). The management of these conditions can be difficult. Nonsteroidal antiinflamatory drugs (NSAIDs) are the first choice but are often not effective. Sulfasalazine has been effective in some cases, and occasionally immunosuppressive agents are indicated, which is problematic in this population. Effective ART is also helpful in treating these inflammatory conditions.[31]

HIV-associated Arthritis

HIV infection is associated with an arthropathy similar to other viruses (eg, hepatitis B). It is typically a transient, nonerosive, oligoarthritis that affects the lower extremities, lasting less than 6 weeks. It can occur at any time during the course of HIV infection. Synovial fluid analysis is noninflammatory. Rheumatoid factor and antinuclear antibodies tests are negative in this condition. The treatment consists of NSAIDs, and the condition tends to be self-limited.[31,32] Painful articular syndrome has been described in patients infected with HIV. It is characterized by an acute onset of severe arthralgia, a self-limited condition that usually lasts less than 24 hours. Like HIV-associated arthropathy, the synovial fluid analysis is unremarkable.[31]

MYOPATHIES
Polymyositis

Polymyositis can occur at any stage of HIV infection. It is an idiopathic inflammatory process of the skeletal muscle.[31,33] Patients present with a subacute, progressive, proximal muscle weakness with an increased creatine kinase level. It may be the first sign of HIV infection. Treatment with corticosteroids seems to be beneficial as it is in other inflammatory myopathies. Medications such as high-dose zidovudine (AZT or ZDV) are associated with a polymyositis-like picture in a small percentage of patients. Zidovudine-induced myopathy is initially clinically indistinguishable from polymyositis. Clinical and laboratory features normalize several months after discontinuing therapy.[29]

Pyomyositis

Pyomyositis is a primary deep muscle abscess seen more often in patients infected with HIV than those with no HIV infection. *Staphylococcus aureus* is the culprit organism in more than 90% of cases.[1] The inciting factor of the infection is unclear. It has been postulated that a transient bacteremia seeds traumatized muscle.[13] The disease is indolent, and initially patients complain of crampy pain along 1 muscle group, with a low-grade fever.[34] It may be difficult to distinguish from polymyositis or other forms of inflammatory muscle disease. Induration may be present. The most common sites of involvement include the quadriceps, the gluteal, and iliopsoas muscles. After 1 to 3 weeks, the pain becomes progressively worse and the fever more pronounced.[10,13] If undiagnosed, the patient will likely become septic. CT scan, MRI, and ultrasound are all helpful in making the diagnosis. MRI is probably more sensitive early in the course before the fluid collection becomes prominent. Treatment is by drainage and systemic antimicrobial therapy directed at *S aureus*.

SUMMARY

Various musculoskeletal manifestations can occur in the individual infected with HIV. The spectrum of disease is a result of a combination of the immunosuppressive effects of the virus, the immune response to the virus, and the medications used to treat the disease. ART has altered the course of the disease and this shift has changed the musculoskeletal manifestations. There are now fewer opportunistic infections and an increase in osteopenia and osteonecrosis.

Patients who are profoundly immunosuppressed are predisposed to disseminated and unusual infections, including disseminated bartonella, tuberculosis, and atypical mycobacterial infections. Noninfectious spondyloarthropathies are also more commonly associated with HIV, as are myopathies. The emergency physician must be aware of these specific manifestations of orthopedic disease in the patient with to increase the likelihood of early diagnosis, treatment, and appropriate referral.

REFERENCES

1. Biviji AA, Paiment GD, Steinbach LS. Musculoskeletal manifestations of human immunodeficiency virus infection. J Am Acad Orthop Surg 2002;10:312–20.

2. Venkat A, Piontkowsky DM, Cooney RR, et al. Care of the HIV-positive patient in the emergency department in the era of highly active antiretorival therapy. Ann Emerg Med 2008;52(3):274–85.
3. The Antiretroviral Therapy Cohort Collaboration. The changing incidence of AIDS events in patients receiving highly active antiretroviral therapy. Arch Intern Med 2005;165:416–23.
4. Glesby MJ. Bone disorders in human immunodeficiency virus infection. Clin Infect Dis 2003;37(Suppl 2):S91–5.
5. Casado E, Olive A, Holgado S, et al. Musculoskeletal manifestations in patients positive for human immunodeficiency virus: correlation with CD4 count. J Rheumatol 2001;28:802–4.
6. Goedert JJ, Cote TR, Virgo P, et al. Spectrum of AIDS-associated malignant disorders. Lancet 1998;351(9119):1833–9.
7. Antman K, Chang Y. Kaposi's sarcoma. N Engl J Med 2000;342(14):1027–38.
8. Krishna G, Chitkara RK. Osseous Kaposi's sarcoma. JAMA 2003;289(9):1106.
9. Isenberger DW, Aronson NE. Lytic vertebral lesions: an unusual manifestation of AIDS-related Kaposi's sarcoma. Clin Infect Dis 1994;19(4):751–5.
10. Moylett EH, Shearer WT. HIV: clinical manifestations. J Allergy Clin Immunol 2002;110(1):3–16.
11. Shafer RW, Edlin BR. Tuberculosis in patients infected with human immunodeficiency virus: perspective on the past decade. Clin Infect Dis 1996;22:683–704.
12. CDC. Targeted tuberculin testing and treatment of latent tuberculosis infection. MMWR 2000;49(No. RR-6):8–9.
13. Tehranzadeh J, Ter-Organesyan RR, Steinbach LS. Musculoskeletal disorders associated with HIV infection and AIDS. Part 1: infectious musculoskeletal conditions. Skeletal Radiol 2004;33:240–59.
14. Barnes PF, Bloch AB, Davidson PT, et al. Tuberculosis in patients with human immunodeficiency virus infection. N Engl J Med 1991;324:1644–50.
15. Jellis JE. Orthopaedic surgery and HIV disease in Africa. Int Orthop 1996;20(4):253–6.
16. Kovacs JA, Masur H. Prophylaxis against opportunistic infections in patients with human immunodeficiency virus infection. N Engl J Med 2000;342(19):1416–29.
17. Hirsch R, Miller SM, Kazi S, et al. Human immunodeficiency virus-associated atypical mycobacterial skeletal infections. Semin Arthritis Rheum 1996;25(5):347–56.
18. Mohle-Boetani JC, Koehler JE, Berger TG, et al. Bacillary angiomatosis and bacillary peliosis in patients infected with human immunodeficiency virus. Clin Infect Dis 1993;17(4):612–24.
19. Paton NI, Macallan DC, Griffen GE, et al. Bone mineral density in patients with human immunodeficiency virus infection. Calcif Tissue Int 1997;61:30–2.
20. Tebas P, Powderly WG, Claxton S, et al. Accelerated bone mineral loss in HIV-infected patients receiving potent antiretroviral therapy. AIDS 2000;1:F63–7.
21. Aberg JA, Kaplan JE, Libman H, et al. Primary care guidelines for the management of persons infected with human immunodeficiency virus: 2009 update by the HIV medicine association of the infectious diseases society of America. Clin Infect Dis 2009;49(5):651–81.
22. Ebeling PR. Osteoporosis in men. N Engl J Med 2008;358(14):1474–82.
23. Brown P, Crane L. Avascular necrosis of bone in patients with human immunodeficiency virus infection: report of 6 cases and review of the literature. Clin Infect Dis 2001;32:1221–6.
24. Lew DP, Waldvogel FA. Osteomyelitis. Lancet 2004;364(9431):369–79.

25. Pineda C, Vargas A, Rodriguez AV. Imaging of osteomyelitis: current concepts. Infect Dis Clin North Am 2006;20:789–825.

26. Zalavras CG, Dellamaggiora R, Patzakis MJ, et al. Septic arthritis in patients with human immunodeficiency virus. Clin Orthop Relat Res 2006;451:46–9.

27. Garcia-De La Torre I. Advances in the management of septic arthritis. Infect Dis Clin North Am 2006;20:773–88.

28. Frazee BW, Fee C, Lambert L. How common is MRSA in adult septic arthritis. Ann Emerg Med 2009;54(5):695–700.

29. Tehranzadeh J, Ter-Organesyan RR, Steinbach LS. Musculoskeletal disorders associated with HIV infection and AIDS. Part 2: non-infectious musculoskeletal conditions. Skeletal radiol 2004;33:311–20.

30. Clark MR, Solinger AM, Hochberg MC. Human immunodeficiency virus infection is not associated with Reiter's syndrome. Data from three large cohort studies. Rheum Dis Clin North Am 1992;18:267–76.

31. Reveille JD, Williams FM. Rheumatologic complications of HIV infection. Best Pract Res Clin Rheumatol 2006;20(6):1159–79.

32. Walker UA, Tyndall A, Daikeler T. Rheumatic conditions in human immunodeficiency virus infection. Rheumatology (Oxford) 2008;47(7):952–9.

33. Dalakas MC, Pezeshkpour GH, Gnavall M, et al. Polymyositis associated with AIDS retrovirus. JAMA 1986;256:2381–3.

34. Schwartzman WA, Lambertus MW, Kennedy CA, et al. Staphylococcal pyomyositis in patients infected by the human immunodeficiency virus. Am J Med 1991;90:595–600.

Renal and Urologic Emergencies in the HIV-infected Patient

Stephen Y. Liang, MD*, E. Turner Overton, MD

KEYWORDS

- Human immunodeficiency virus • AIDS • Acute renal failure
- Chronic kidney disease • Urologic emergencies

Over the last 2 decades, the introduction of antiretroviral therapy (ART) has dramatically improved morbidity and mortality from human immunodeficiency virus (HIV).[1,2] Although opportunistic infections still abound in populations with poor access or adherence to care, the spectrum of disease in treatment-adherent HIV patients has shifted toward chronic medical problems frequently associated with end-organ damage, medication toxicity, and other causes unrelated to HIV or acquired immunodeficiency syndrome (AIDS).[3,4] In the modern era of ART, renal disease has become a well-recognized consequence of both HIV infection and therapy.[5,6] This article discusses aspects of renal and urologic disorders unique to the HIV-infected patient presenting to the emergency department (ED). A broad survey of the differential diagnosis and management of acute and chronic renal failure in the HIV-infected patient as well as a review of selected urological emergencies is presented. Within this context, it is hoped that the emergency physician will better appreciate the special considerations necessary to provide appropriate care for HIV-infected patients with renal and urological emergencies.

ACUTE RENAL FAILURE IN HIV

Acute renal failure (ARF), or acute kidney injury, is defined as a sudden decline in glomerular filtration rate, leading to the net retention of metabolic waste products. Subsequent derangements in fluid and serum electrolyte balance may lead to volume overload, hyperkalemia, and metabolic acidosis requiring emergent medical intervention and even hemodialysis. Apart from oliguria or anuria, the symptoms of ARF may be nonspecific. The diagnosis is usually confirmed by laboratory evaluation. An increase in serum creatinine or blood urea nitrogen (BUN) concentration, the latter of which is termed azotemia, is usually apparent in ARF, but may be absent in its early

Division of Infectious Diseases, Washington University School of Medicine, 660 South Euclid Avenue, Campus Box 8051, Saint Louis, MO 63110-1093, USA
* Corresponding author.
E-mail address: sliang@dom.wustl.edu

Emerg Med Clin N Am 28 (2010) 343–354
doi:10.1016/j.emc.2010.01.010
0733-8627/10/$ – see front matter © 2010 Elsevier Inc. All rights reserved.

emed.theclinics.com

stages. Generally accepted laboratory criteria for ARF include a 50% reduction in creatinine clearance or a 50% increase in serum creatinine level above baseline.

ARF remains a common disease of the HIV-infected patient in the era of ART. A study of adult hospitalized HIV-infected patients in New York State found that the incidence of ARF rose from 2.9% in 1995 (pre-ART) to 6% in 2003 (post-ART).[7] This change was compared with a less dramatic increase from 1.0% to 2.7% in non-HIV–infected patients. Risk factors for ARF included older age, male gender, diabetes mellitus, chronic kidney disease, and liver disease. ARF in HIV-infected patients was also associated with a 27% in-hospital mortality, a sixfold increase when compared with HIV-infected patients without ARF in 2003 (odds ratio: 5.83; 95% confidence interval: 5.11–6.65). In the critically ill inpatient HIV population with multiorgan failure, overall mortality of patients with ARF may be as high as 43.3%.[8] ARF occurred more frequently in men, patients coinfected with hepatitis C, and those with advanced HIV, as evidenced by lower $CD4^+$ cell counts (<200 cells/mm^3), higher HIV RNA levels (>10,000 copies/mL), and previous AIDS-defining illness. A subsequent analysis using the same cohort demonstrated a dose-response pattern linking lower $CD4^+$ cell counts with a higher incidence of ARF.[9]

The differential diagnosis for ARF in HIV-infected patients presenting to the ED can be broken down into 3 broad categories: prerenal, intrinsic, and postobstructive (**Box 1**). Within these categories, prerenal azotemia, ischemic and nephrotoxic acute tubular necrosis (ATN), acute interstitial nephritis (AIN), crystal-induced nephropathy, and obstructive uropathy are significant etiologies for ARF with unique considerations in the setting of HIV and ART. Of note, medications have been implicated in up to a third of all cases of ARF in HIV-infected patients.[10] In most cases however, the etiology of ARF is multifactorial.

Prerenal Azotemia

Prerenal azotemia accounts for as much as 40% of ARF in hospitalized HIV-infected patients.[11] Both true and effective volume depletion lead to renal hypoperfusion, precipitating ARF. True volume depletion, or hypovolemia, may frequently be secondary to gastrointestinal fluid losses from vomiting or diarrhea, which may suggest an infection, a medication side effect, or a myriad of other diseases. Poor oral intake related to anorexia, dysphagia, or odynophagia may compound volume deficits. Fever and tachypnea may account for significant insensible fluid losses. Endocrinologic disorders such as adrenal insufficiency and isolated hypoaldosteronism may cause

---

Box 1
Causes of acute renal failure in the HIV-infected patient

Prerenal

    Prerenal azotemia

Intrinsic

    Acute tubular necrosis (ischemic vs nephrotoxic)

    Acute interstitial nephritis

    Crystal-induced nephropathy

Postobstructive

    Crystal-induced nephropathy

    Nephrolithiasis

urinary sodium wasting, leading to dehydration. Likewise, disordered water regulation from central or nephrogenic diabetes insipidus may lead to profound volume depletion. Diuretics used to treat conditions such as liver failure and cirrhosis may also bring about significant hypovolemia.

Effective volume depletion stemming from euvolemic or hypervolemic states found in sepsis, congestive heart failure, or cirrhosis may result in renal hypoperfusion and subsequent prerenal azotemia. In sepsis, a systemic inflammatory response to infection leads to endotoxin-mediated vasodilatation, arterial hypotension, and organ hypoperfusion. The use of vasopressors to treat hypotension may further worsen organ and specifically renal perfusion. In congestive heart failure and cirrhosis, low cardiac output and third-spacing of fluid are responsible for intravascular volume depletion and hence renal hypoperfusion. Similarly, third-spacing in severe pancreatitis may also lead to effective volume depletion and ARF.

The appropriate management of prerenal azotemia depends on the underlying cause. While true volume depletion requires aggressive hydration, the source, whether infectious, gastrointestinal, endocrinologic, or iatrogenic, should be addressed as part of the comprehensive workup. A patient with ARF from sepsis may not only require aggressive hydration but timely antibiotic and vasopressor therapy, recognizing that ARF may worsen and necessitate hemodialysis. In contrast, the patient with congestive heart disease from HIV cardiomyopathy and prerenal azotemia may require preload and afterload reduction with nitrates and an angiotensin-converting enzyme inhibitor, followed by diuretics. In severely decompensated patients, inotropic support may be indicated. The management of ARF in the HIV-infected patient with cirrhosis or the hepatorenal syndrome requires interventions to address portal hypertension (eg, octreotide, midodrine, vasopressin analogues, transjugular intrahepatic portosystemic shunt, transplantation) and decreased plasma oncotic pressure (eg, albumin). These decisions should be made in consultation with an intensivist, hepatologist, and nephrologist on admission. The treatment of severe pancreatitis may require not only aggressive hydration but also discontinuation of offending drugs and evaluation for biliary tract obstruction.

Acute Tubular Necrosis

Ischemic and nephrotoxic acute tubular necrosis are common causes of intrinsic ARF, accounting for 26% to 46% of all cases of ARF in HIV-infected patients.[10,12] In both forms, ATN is manifest by renal epithelial damage leading to sloughing, cast formation within the renal tubule, and finally ARF. Classically, "muddy brown" coarse granular casts may be seen in the urine sediment. Ischemic ATN represents the severe end of the spectrum of hypoperfusion injury opposite prerenal azotemia. Ischemic ATN is most frequently associated with severe hypovolemia, particularly in sepsis, as previously mentioned. Mortality in AIDS patients from ischemic ATN is historically high, given the likelihood of multiple organ dysfunction in the setting of sepsis.[12,13]

Nephrotoxic ATN may occur with renal tubular exposure to medications, exogenous toxins, hemoglobin, and myoglobin. Nephrotoxic ATN may result from the use of nonsteroidal anti-inflammatory drugs (NSAIDs) as well as a host of antimicrobial agents. Aminoglycosides including gentamicin, tobramycin, and amikacin are known to cause ATN. Likewise, amphotericin B and pentamidine, which are still employed to treat refractory cases of *Pneumocystis jirovechi* pneumonia and cryptococcal infection, are also well-known nephrotoxic agents.[11] Cidofovir and forscarnet, 2 agents used to treat resistant cytomegalovirus infections, have been associated with ATN. Tenofovir, a nucleotide reverse transcriptase inhibitor, may cause proximal tubular dysfunction leading to acidosis, nephrotic-range proteinuria, and ATN.[14] Injury from tenofovir may be augmented particularly when it is used in conjunction with a boosted protease inhibitor (eg, low-dose ritonavir) to increase serum levels of tenofovir.[15] Rhabdomyolysis in HIV-infected patients may lead to ATN, particularly when triggered by infection, trauma, or substance abuse (eg, cocaine, heroin, alcohol).[13,16] Of particular importance to the emergency physician, intravenous radiocontrast may also inflict direct tubular injury leading to contrast-induced nephropathy.

Management of ATN requires volume repletion until the patient is euvolemic. Nephrotoxic agents should be promptly discontinued. The use of further nephrotoxic agents including intravenous radiocontrast should be avoided when possible.

Acute Interstitial Nephritis

Acute interstitial nephritis frequently results from a hypersensitivity reaction to a medication involving the renal tubules and interstitium, leading to ARF. Trimethoprim-sulfamethoxazole (TMP-SMX), allopurinol, phenytoin, and rifampin have been identified as common causes of AIN in HIV-infected patients.[11,13] β-Lactam antibiotics, quinolones, and NSAIDs have also traditionally been associated with AIN in the general population. Although a history of fever, rash, and eosinophilia preceded by initiation of a new medication may guide diagnosis, a causative drug for AIN is frequently undeterminable, especially in the setting of polypharmacy. Management of AIN focuses on discontinuation of the offending agent and supportive care.

Crystal-induced Nephropathy

Crystal-induced nephropathy occurs when a medication precipitates out of the urine as crystals in the renal tubule, causing obstruction. Volume depletion and low urinary flow likely further promote crystal formation. Sulfadiazine, used to treat cerebral toxoplasmosis, has historically been associated with crystalluria.[17] Likewise, indinavir, atazanavir, and foscarnet have all been known to cause crystal nephropathy.[18–20] Intravenous acyclovir, frequently used for empirical coverage of herpes simplex virus (HSV) encephalitis, carries a risk of crystal-induced nephropathy as well. Aside from medications, crystal-induced nephropathy may be seen in conditions associated with hyperuricemia. In particular, spontaneous or chemotherapy-related tumor lysis syndrome in the setting of AIDS-associated lymphoma may promote hyperuricosuria and subsequent crystal deposition, leading to ARF.

Appropriate management of crystal-induced nephropathy entails aggressive fluid resuscitation to clear the crystals obstructing the tubular lumen and discontinuation of the offending medication. Dose adjustment of intravenous acyclovir in the setting of preexisting chronic kidney disease, avoidance of rapid bolus infusion, and adequate hydration to ensure a euvolemic state prior to administration may help prevent acyclovir crystalluria.[21] In tumor lysis syndrome, aggressive hydration remains the mainstay. In severe cases, rasburicase, a urate oxidase, may be indicated to hasten renal elimination of uric acid.

Obstructive Uropathy

Although less common, obstructive uropathy in the HIV-infected patient may be responsible for as much as 17% of cases of ARF in some studies.[12] Ureterocalyceal obstruction may occur as a consequence of urolithiasis, blood clots, extrinsic compression of the ureters from retroperitoneal lymphadenopathy (as in AIDS-associated lymphoma, disseminated histoplasmosis, or *Mycobacterium avium complex*), or fibrosis from radiation therapy. In addition to stones and clots, urethral obstruction may result from benign prostatic hypertrophy or stricture, leading to significant urinary retention. Fungal collections of *Candida albicans* and *Aspergillus* can also lead to obstruction. In severe cases of obstruction, ureteral stenting or nephrostomy may be necessary to decompress and drain the kidney.

Urolithiasis is a known complication of therapy with the protease inhibitor indinavir. More than 20% of the drug is unmetabolized and excreted in the urine, leading to crystal formation when the urine pH is greater than 6.[22] As much as 8% of HIV-infected patients taking indinavir may develop urologic symptoms consistent with urolithiasis or crystalluria.[18] Renal colic with indinavir stones or crystalluria is marked by classic symptoms such as dysuria, urgency, flank pain, and hematuria.[18] Indinivar stones are radiolucent and usually not visualized on routine imaging modalities such as abdominal radiography or computed tomography.[23] The management of indinavir urolithiasis remains conservative, emphasizing adequate hydration and pain control. Atazanavir, another protease inhibitor, has also been reported to cause urolithiasis by a similar mechanism.[24]

Chronic Kidney Disease in HIV

In addition to ARF, the emergency physician is likely to take care of HIV-infected patients with underlying renal disease, either from HIV-associated nephropathy or chronic kidney disease related to other comorbid illnesses.

HIV-Associated Nephropathy

HIV-associated nephropathy (HIVAN) was first described during the early stages of the HIV epidemic during the 1980s before the advent of ART. From 1982 to 1986, Rao and colleagues[25] described 78 patients with AIDS at 2 New York City hospitals who required evaluation for renal disease. Of these patients, 30% had reversible ARF, secondary to nephrotoxic or ischemic injury. The remainder developed proteinuria and azotemia, rapidly progressing to end-stage renal disease (ESRD) despite hemodialysis. Only 2 patients in this latter group survived beyond 6 months of initial presentation. This novel illness, later recognized as HIVAN, was characterized by nephrotic-range proteinuria (>3.5 g/d), focal and segmental glomerulosclerosis on renal biopsy, and a rapidly fatal course.

HIVAN has a prevalence ranging from 3.5% to 12%, and remains the third leading cause of ESRD in African Americans aged 20 to 64 years.[26] Host factors such as race and family history play an important part in determining a patient's susceptibility to developing HIVAN. African American HIV-infected individuals with a family history of ESRD are more than 5 times as likely to develop HIVAN as similar individuals without a family history.[27] In contrast to classic nephrotic disease, peripheral edema and hypertension are frequently absent in HIVAN despite marked proteinuria.[28]

HIVAN remains a disease of late HIV and AIDS, with the greatest rates reported in patients with CD4+ cell count of less than 200 cells/mm^3 and HIV RNA levels greater than 100,000 copies/mL.[29] Medical management of HIVAN includes the early initiation of angiotensin-converting enzyme inhibitors, glucocorticoids, and most importantly, ART. Whereas survival from HIVAN was once measured in months, HIV-infected patients with HIVAN successfully treated with ART now enjoy survival measured in years, often with significant improvement in their renal function. In a clinical cohort of 3976 HIV-infected patients seen at Johns Hopkins Hospital between 1989 and 2001, the risk of HIVAN was reduced by 60% with the implementation of ART.[30]

Chronic Kidney Disease

As HIV-infected patients live longer, the risk of chronic kidney disease (CKD) has increased substantially. Risk factors for CKD in HIV-infected patients parallel those of the general population. Age and comorbid illnesses such as diabetes mellitus and hypertension confer a greater risk of CKD. In fact, the incidence of diabetes mellitus in HIV-infected men on ART has been demonstrated to be greater than 4 times that of HIV-negative men in the Multicenter AIDS Cohort Study.[31] CKD disproportionately affects African Americans. In a study of US veterans, the incidence of ESRD among HIV-infected African American patients was nearly 10 times higher than that of HIV-infected white patients and similar to that of non-HIV–infected African Americans with diabetes mellitus.[32] Likewise, Lucas and colleagues[29] have reported that the prevalence of CKD in HIV-infected patients increased from 47.7 per 1000 in the pre-ART era to 69.3 per 1000 people in the ART era, owing in part to improved survival rates with aggressive antiretroviral and renal therapies. Indeed, survival rates of HIV-infected hemodialysis patients has improved significantly since the advent of ART, although they have yet to approach that of non-HIV–infected patients.[33] In selected instances, HIV-infected patients on ART with CKD may even be candidates for renal transplantation.

The HIV-infected patient with CKD presenting to the ED is likely to have many of the same problems and emergencies seen in non-HIV–infected CKD patients. Noncompliance with dietary and fluid intake as well as missed hemodialysis may lead to worsening uremia and volume overload. Uremia may precipitate encephalopathy, pericarditis, and bleeding diastheses. Volume overload may result in pulmonary edema, congestive heart failure, and hypertensive crises. Hemodialysis, in and of itself, may be complicated by hypotension from excessive fluid removal. Hemodialysis catheters may become infected. Although hemodialysis catheter-related bacteremia is equally likely in HIV-infected and non-HIV–infected patients, the clinical course in HIV-infected patients is often more severe, with a greater chance of polymicrobial infection.[34] Vascular grafts and arteriovenous fistulas may become thrombosed or stenosed, or conversely may produce life-threatening hemorrhage.

UROLOGIC EMERGENCIES IN HIV

HIV-infected patients are at heightened risk for several urologic emergencies, many of which are infectious in etiology (**Box 2**). Infection may occur anywhere along the urinary tract and tends to affect AIDS patients disproportionately, given their profound immunosuppression. Much of the existing literature describing urologic disease in HIV-infected patients comes from the early years of the AIDS epidemic in the 1980s and early 1990s. Although the initial approach and management of these illnesses in the ED does not differ greatly from that of the non-HIV–infected patient, it is important to recognize certain aspects of these urologic infections that may be unique to the HIV-infected patient.

Urinary tract infections (UTIs) are commonly encountered in the HIV-infected patient, particularly when the CD4$^+$ cell count is less than 200 cells/mm^3 or the viral load is high.[35–37] In the pre-ART era, UTIs were diagnosed in anywhere from 6% to 20% of AIDS patients.[38–40] Dysuria, urinary frequency, urgency, fever, and suprapubic pain are common presenting symptoms. In one study, *Enterococcus* spp, *Escherichia coli*, and *Pseudomonas aeruginosa* were found to be the most commonly isolated organisms.[41] Other infecting bacteria included *Klebsiella pneumoniae*, *Proteus* spp, *Enterobacter* spp, *Staphylococcus* spp, *Serratia* spp, and *Salmonella* spp. In patients with AIDS, atypical infections with fungi (eg, *Candida albicans*, *Aspergillus fumigatus*, *Cryptococcus neoformans, Pneumocystis jirovecii*), mycobacteria (eg, *Mycobacterium tuberculosis* and *Mycobacterium avium-intracellulare*), and viruses (eg, cytomegalovirus and adenovirus) are also possible. While empirical antibiotics are indicated for the treatment of symptomatic UTIs, a urine culture should be obtained before initiation

---

Box 2
Common urologic conditions in HIV-infected patients

Kidney

    Pyelonephritis

    Renal abscess

    Urolithiasis

Ureter

    Obstruction by retroperitoneal lymphadenopathy (eg, malignancy, infection)

Bladder

    Urinary tract infection

Prostate

    Prostatitis

    Prostatic abscess

Urethra

    Urethritis

Scrotum

    Epididymitis/orchitis

    Abscess

    Fournier gangrene

External genitalia

    Genital ulcer disease

---

of therapy to confirm antibiotic sensitivity. High rates of antimicrobial resistance have been reported, as HIV-infected patients are more likely to be on prophylactic antibiotics (eg, TMP-SMX) against opportunistic infection, and are frequently exposed to a broad range of empirical antibiotics in the advanced stages of their disease.[42] A fluoroquinolone (eg, ciprofloxacin) is generally first-line empirical therapy for an uncomplicated UTI. HIV-infected patients with UTIs may require longer durations of antimicrobial therapy depending on the organism involved and are more likely to experience recurrence. UTI in the HIV-infected patient also has the potential to progress to pyelonephritis, bacteremia, and sepsis.

Renal abscesses, particularly from systemic fungal infections (*C albicans, Aspergillus*) and disseminated tuberculosis, may also be seen.[43,44] *Staphylococcus aureus* remains the causative organism in most cases. Hematogenous spread from an extrarenal source to the kidney is typically the primary cause of renal abscesses. Symptoms can include fever, chills, nausea, vomiting, abdominal pain, and flank pain. Computed tomography and ultrasound are important tools for establishing the diagnosis. Blood and urine cultures are important in guiding antibiotic therapy. Percutaneous abscess drainage and even nephrectomy may be necessary as adjuncts to broad-spectrum antibiotic therapy and fluid resuscitation.

According to a study from the pre-ART era in 1989, the prevalence of bacterial prostatitis among HIV-infected patients was 3% in asymptomatic individuals, increasing to 14% in patients with AIDS.[45] Prostatitis is usually heralded by dysuria, frequency, urgency, fever, and perineal pain, coupled with an enlarged and tender prostate on digital rectal examination. Bacteriuria may be present on urine microscopy. Whereas infections secondary to *E coli* and other gram-negative bacteria are most common, atypical infection with fungi, mycobacteria, and viruses are also possible. In men younger than 35 years, *Neisseria gonorrhoeae* and *Chlamydia trachomatis* are responsible for a majority of cases. Treatment with one dose of intramuscular ceftriaxone followed by a 10-day course of doxycycline is appropriate. *E coli* is a more common cause in men older than 35 years and requires a 2-week course of oral fluoroquinolone (eg, ciprofloxacin). HIV-infected men are at higher risk for chronic prostatitis as well as developing prostatic abscesses in the setting of relapsing infection, which may require not only longer durations of antibiotic therapy but also surgical drainage.

Immunosuppression is a known risk factor for necrotizing Fournier gangrene and fasciitis of the scrotum and perineum, particularly in the setting of comorbid diabetes mellitus or alcoholism.[46] Although rare, Fournier gangrene has been reported in HIV-infected patients and constitutes a urologic emergency. *E coli*, *Bacteroides* spp, *Streptococci*, *Staphylococci*, *Peptostreptococcus* spp, and *Clostridium* spp have all been implicated in this polymicrobial infection of the subcutaneous tissues that subsequently tracks along fascial planes.[47] Patients with Fournier gangrene may present with fever and perineal pain. Erythema, induration, tenderness, and crepitus may be noted in the perineum, and the affected area may appear necrotic. The risk of progressing to bacteremia, sepsis, and hemodynamic collapse is great. The diagnosis is clinical. Initial management should include aggressive fluid resuscitation and broad-spectrum antibiotic therapy to cover gram-positive, gram-negative, and anaerobic organisms. Prompt surgical debridement is the definitive treatment. Recent estimates of mortality from Fournier gangrene in the general population approach 7.5%, although older case series have reported mortality as high as 20% to 40%.[48]

As in the general population, HIV-infected patients are at risk for acquiring sexually transmitted infections when engaged in risky sexual practices. Male urethritis typically stems from infection with *N gonorrhoeae* or *C trachomatis*. Empirical treatment should cover both organisms, given that as many as 50% of patients may be coinfected. Gonococcal infection is typically treated with a single dose of intramuscular ceftriaxone, whereas chlamydial infection is covered by a single oral dose of azithromycin or a week-long course of doxycycline. The use of fluoroquinolones is not recommended, given antibiotic resistance patterns in gonorrhea. Epididymitis may result from an untreated urethritis or UTI. Causative organisms and initial treatment approach parallel those of acute prostatitis. In men younger than 35 years, *N gonorrhoeae* and *C trachomatis* are treated with a dose of intramuscular ceftriaxone followed by a 10-day course of doxycycline. In those older than 35 years, the more common *E coli* infection is treated with a 2-week course of an oral fluoroquinolone (eg, ciprofloxacin). Untreated epididymitis can lead to abscess formation, particularly in atypical infections involving *Candida*, cytomegalovirus, mycobacteria, *Toxoplasmosis*, or *Salmonella*.

Genital ulcer disease in the HIV-infected patient can be caused by sexually transmitted infections such as genital herpes, syphilis, and chancroid. Herpes simplex virus type 2 (HSV-2) affects 50% to 90% of HIV-1-infected patients.[49] The clinical presentation of genital herpes in HIV-infected patients can range anywhere from small fissures to extensive, painful, and necrotic ulcerations in severe disease. Episodic treatment is no different from that of the general population and may consist of acyclovir, famciclovir, or valacyclovir. Genital herpes outbreaks are slower to respond to therapy in HIV-infected patients, particularly in those with lower CD4+ cell counts, and may require anywhere from 5 to 14 days to clear.[49] Up to 5% of HSV infections in HIV-infected patients may be resistant to acyclovir, compared with less than 1% in the general population.[50] These infections are likely to be resistant to famciclovir and vala-cyclovir as well, and may require intravenous foscarnet.[49]

Syphilis remains a significant cause of genital ulcer disease in the HIV-infected patient. Coinfection with syphilis has been known to increase HIV viral load and decrease CD4[+] cell count.[51] The natural progression of syphilis is not significantly changed in the HIV-infected patient. Primary syphilis is marked by the development of a painless ulcer (chancre) on a mucosal surface, most commonly the genitalia or anus, from a few weeks to several months after exposure. These lesions are highly infectious. HIV-infected patients with primary syphilis tend to present more frequently with multiple ulcers compared with noninfected patients.[52] A classic diffuse maculo-papular rash that may involve the palms and soles marks the secondary stage, and may be accompanied by fever, malaise, arthralgias, myalgias, and lymphadenopathy. Condylomata lata are wartlike lesions that may occur on the genitalia or near the anus during this stage. Primary and secondary syphilis may overlap more frequently in HIV-infected patients, resulting in a presentation of chancres concurrently with a rash.[52] As in the non-HIV population, treatment of early syphilis in HIV consists of a single dose of intramuscular benzathine penicillin G. Some have recommended treating HIV-infected patients with primary or secondary syphilis with 3 doses of benzathine penicillin G at weekly intervals. Of note, HIV-infected patients presenting with early syphilis may be at greater risk of developing neurosyphilis.[53] Neurologic complaints such as head-ache, stiff neck, visual and hearing changes, and focal weakness should prompt lumbar puncture and further inpatient evaluation.

More common in developing countries, chancroid is manifest by painful lesions on the genitalia with tender inguinal lymphadenopathy. Infection with *Haemophilus ducreyi*, the etiologic organism of chancroid, is effectively treated with a single oral dose of azithromycin or a single intramuscular dose of ceftriaxone. HIV-infected patients with chancroid are more likely to fail initial therapy and frequently require longer durations of treatment. While usually nonemergent, sexually transmitted infec-tions leading to urethritis, cervicitis, and genital ulcer disease in the HIV-infected patient may increase a patient's risk of transmitting HIV to other individuals through increased risk of viral shedding from genital mucosal surfaces and ulcerations.[54] Advice on adequate antibiotic therapy and safe sexual practices must be reinforced to the patient. The emergency physician's public health contribution to helping prevent the spread of HIV in the community cannot be overemphasized, even in the busy environment of the ED.

SUMMARY

As frontline medical providers, emergency physicians are integral in the acute care of HIV-infected patients. Direct organ injury from HIV infection, concomitant immunosup-pression, and medication-related complications of contemporary therapy ensure that HIV-infected patients are at risk for a wide spectrum of renal and urologic emergen-cies, distinct in many ways from those of the general population. Frequent etiologies of ARF may include prerenal azotemia, ischemic or nephrotoxic ATN, acute interstitial nephritis, crystal-induced nephropathy, or obstructive uropathy. Chronic renal failure may result directly from HIVAN or from long-standing hypertension or diabetes melli-tus. HIV-infected patients may be at greater risk for developing UTIs, renal abscesses, and other illnesses affecting the genitourinary tract. It is hoped that a better under-standing of these disease processes within the context of the HIV-infected patient will enable the emergency physician to better care for this complex and rapidly growing patient population.

REFERENCES

1. Palella FJ, Delaney KM, Moorman AC, et al. Declining morbidity and mortality among patients with advanced human immunodeficiency virus infection. N Engl J Med 1998;338(13):853–60.
2. Detels R, Munoz A, McFarlane G, et al. Effectiveness of potent antiretroviral therapy on time to AIDS and death in men with known HIV infection duration. JAMA 1998;280(17):1497–503.
3. Palella FJ, Baker RK, Moorman AC, et al. Mortality in the highly active antiretroviral therapy era: changing causes of death and disease in the HIV outpatient study. J Acquir Immune Defic Syndr 2006;43(1):27–34.
4. Lau B, Gange SJ, Moore RD. Risk of non-AIDS-related mortality may exceed risk of AIDS-related mortality among individuals enrolling into care with CD4+ counts greater than 200 cells/mm^3. J Acquir Immune Defic Syndr 2007;44(2):179–87.
5. Selik RM, Byers RH, Dworkin MS. Trends in diseases reported on US death certificates that mentioned HIV infection, 1987–1999. J Acquir Immune Defic Syndr 2002;29(4):378–87.
6. Schwartz EJ, Szczech LA, Ross MJ, et al. Highly active antiretroviral therapy and the epidemic of HIV+ end-stage renal disease. J Am Soc Nephrol 2005;16: 2412–20.
7. Wyatt CM, Arons RR, Klotman PE, et al. Acute renal failure in hospitalized patients with HIV: risk factors and impact on in-hospital mortality. AIDS 2006;20(4):561–5.
8. Lopes JA, Fernandes J, Jorge S, et al. An assessment of the RIFLE criteria for acute renal failure in critically ill HIV-infected patients. Crit Care 2007;11:401–2.
9. Franceschini N, Napravnik S, Finn WF, et al. Immunosuppression, hepatitis C infection, and acute renal failure in HIV-infected patients. J Acquir Immune Defic Syndr 2006;42(3):368–72.
10. Franceschini N, Napravnik S, Eron JJ, et al. Incidence and etiology of acute renal failure among ambulatory HIV-infected patients. Kidney Int 2005;67:1526–31.
11. Valeria A, Neusy AJ. Acute and chronic renal disease in hospitalized AIDS patients. Clin Nephrol 1991;35:110–8.
12. Peraldi MN, Maslo C, Akposso K, et al. Acute renal failure in the course of HIV infection: a single-institution retrospective study of ninety-two patients and sixty renal biopsies. Nephrol Dial Transplant 1999;14:1578–85.
13. Rao TK, Friedman EA. Outcome of severe acute renal failure in patients with acquired immunodeficiency syndrome. Am J Kidney Dis 1995;25:390–8.
14. Coca S, Perazella MA. Rapid communication: acute renal failure associated with tenofovir: evidence of drug-induced nephrotoxicity. Am J Med Sci 2002;324(6): 342–4.
15. Goicoechea M, Liu S, Best B, et al. Greater tenofovir-associated renal function decline with protease inhibitor-based versus nonnucleoside reverse-transcriptase inhibitor-based therapy. J Infect Dis 2008;197:102–8.
16. Joshi MK, Liu HH. Acute rhabdomyolysis and renal failure in HIV-infected patients: risk factors, presentation, and pathophysiology. AIDS Patient Care STDS 2000;14(10):541–8.
17. Dong BJ, Rodriguez RA, Goldschmidt RH. Sulfadiazine-induced crystalluria and renal failure in a patient with AIDS. J Am Board Fam Pract 1999;12(3):243–8.
18. Kopp JB, Miller KD, Mican JM, et al. Crystalluria and urinary tract abnormalities associated with indinavir. Ann Intern Med 1997;127(2):119–25.
19. Izzedine H, M'rad MB, Bardier A, et al. Atazanvir crystal nephropathy. AIDS 2007; 21(17):2357–8.

20. Maurice-Estepa L, Daudon M, Katlama C, et al. Identification of crystals in kidneys of AIDS patients treated with foscarnet. Am J Kidney Dis 1998;32(3): 392–400.
21. Perazella MA. Drug-induced renal failure: update on new medications and unique mechanisms of nephrotoxicity. Am J Med Sci 2003;325(6):349–62.
22. Witte M, Tobon A, Gruenenfelder R, et al. Anuria and acute renal failure resulting from indinavir sulfate induced nephrolithiasis. J Urol 1998;159:498–9.
23. Schwartz BF, Schenkman N, Armenakas NA, et al. Imaging characteristics of indinavir calculi. J Urol 1999;161:1085–7.
24. Chang HR, Pella PM. Atazanavir urolithiasis. N Engl J Med 2006;355(20):2158–9.
25. Rao TK, Friedman EA, Nicastri AD. The types of renal disease in the acquired immunodeficiency syndrome. N Engl J Med 1987;316(17):1062–8.
26. Ross MJ, Klotman PE. Recent progress in HIV-associated nephropathy. J Am Soc Nephrol 2002;13:2997–3004.
27. Freedman BI, Soucie JM, Stone SM, et al. Familial clustering of end-stage renal disease in blacks with HIV-associated nephropathy. Am J Kidney Dis 1999;34: 254–8.
28. Bourgoignie JJ, Meneses R, Ortiz C, et al. The clinical spectrum of renal disease associated with human immunodeficiency virus. Am J Kidney Dis 1988;12:131–7.
29. Lucas GM, Mehta SH, Atta MG, et al. End-stage renal disease and chronic kidney disease in a cohort of African-American HIV-infected and at-risk HIV-seronegative participants followed between 1988 and 2004. AIDS 2007;21:2435–43.
30. Lucas GM, Eustace JA, Sozio S, et al. Highly active antiretroviral therapy and the incidence of HIV-1-associated nephropathy: a 12-year cohort study. AIDS 2004; 18:541–6.
31. Brown TT, Cole SR, Li X, et al. Antiretroviral therapy and the prevalence and incidence of diabetes mellitus in the multicenter AIDS cohort study. Arch Intern Med 2005;165:1179–84.
32. Choi AI, Rodriguez RA, Bacchetti P, et al. Racial differences in end-stage renal disease rates in HIV infection versus diabetes. J Am Soc Nephrol 2007;18: 2968–74.
33. Ahuja TS, Grady J, Khan S. Changing trends in the survival of dialysis patients with human immunodeficiency virus in the United States. J Am Soc Nephrol 2002;13:1889–93.
34. Mitchell D, Krishnasami Z, Allon M. Catheter-related bacteraemia in haemodialysis patients with HIV infection. Nephrol Dial Transplant 2006;21:3185–8.
35. Hoepelman AI, van Buren M, van den Broek J, et al. Bacteriuria in men infected with HIV-1 is related to their immune status (CD4+ cell count). AIDS 1992;6(2): 179–84.
36. Evans JK, McOwan A, Hillman RJ, et al. Incidence of symptomatic urinary tract infections in HIV seropositive patients and the use of cotrimoxazole as prophylaxis against Pneumocystis carinii pneumonia. Genitourin Med 1995;71(2):120–2.
37. Park JC, Buono D, Smith DK, et al. Urinary tract infections in women with or at risk for human immunodeficiency virus infection. Am J Obstet Gynecol 2002;187: 581–8.
38. Kaplan MS, Wechsler M, Benson MC. Urologic manifestations of AIDS. Urology 1987;30(5):441–3.
39. Miles MJ, Melser M, Farah R, et al. The urological manifestations of the acquired immunodeficiency syndrome. J Urol 1989;142:771–3.

40. De Pinho AM, Lopes GS, Ramos-Filho CF, et al. Urinary tract infection in men with AIDS. Genitourin Med 1994;70:30–4.
41. Schönwald S, Begovac J, Skerk V. Urinary tract infections in HIV disease. Int J Antimicrob Agents 1999;11:309–11.
42. Vignesh R, Shankar EM, Murugavel KG, et al. Urinary tract infections due to multi-drug-resistant *Escherichia coli* among persons with HIV disease at a tertiary AIDS care centre in South India. Nephron Clin Pract 2008;110:c55–7.
43. Oosten AW, Sprenger HG, Van Leeuwen JT, et al. Bilateral renal aspergillosis in a patient with AIDS: a case report and review of reported cases. AIDS Patient Care STDS 2008;22(1):1–6.
44. Figueiredo AA, Lucon AM, Júnior RF, et al. Urogenital tuberculosis in immuno-compromised patients. Int Urol Nephrol 2009;41:327–33.
45. Leport C, Rousseau F, Perronne C, et al. Bacterial prostatitis in patients infected with the human immunodeficiency virus. J Urol 1989;141(2):334–6.
46. Bhatnagar AM, Mohite PN, Suthar M. Fournier's gangrene: review of 110 cases for aetiology, predisposing conditions, microorganisms, and modalities for coverage of necrosed scrotum with bare testes. N Z Med J 2008;121:46–56.
47. Merino E, Boix V, Portilla J, et al. Fournier's gangrene in HIV-infected patients. Eur J Clin Microbiol Infect Dis 2001;20:910–3.
48. Sorensen MD, Krieger JN, Rivara FP, et al. Fournier's gangrene: population based epidemiology and outcomes. J Urol 2009;181(5):2120–6.
49. Strick LB, Wald A, Celum C. Management of herpes simplex virus type 2 infection in HIV type 1-infected persons. Clin Infect Dis 2006;43:347–56.
50. Reyes M, Shaik NS, Graber JM, et al. Acyclovir-resistant genital herpes among persons attending sexually transmitted disease and human immunodeficiency virus clinics. Arch Intern Med 2003;163:76–80.
51. Buchacz K, Patel P, Taylor M, et al. Syphilis increases HIV viral load and decreases CD4 cell counts in HIV-infected patients with new syphilis infections. AIDS 2004;18(15):2075–9.
52. Rompalo AM, Joesoef MR, O'Donnell JA, et al. Clinical manifestations of early syphilis by HIV status and gender: results of the syphilis and HIV study. Sex Transm Dis 2001;28(3):158–65.
53. Flood JM, Weinstock HS, Guroy ME, et al. Neurosyphilis during the AIDS epidemic, San Francisco, 1985–1992. J Infect Dis 1998;177(4):931–40.
54. Fleming DT, Wasserheit JN. From epidemiological synergy to public health policy and practice: the contribution of other sexually transmitted diseases to sexual transmission of HIV infection. Sex Transm Infect 1999;75(1):3–17.

Dermatology of the Patient with HIV

Mariam M. Khambaty, MD[a],*, Sam S. Hsu, MD[b]

KEYWORDS

- Dermatology • Rash • HIV • Emergency medicine

Cutaneous diseases affect most patients infected with human immunodeficiency virus (HIV) at some point during their infection. These patients have up to 15 times higher visit rates for common infectious and inflammatory skin conditions than patients not infected with HIV.[1] Although antiretroviral therapy (ART) has decreased the incidence of some rashes, particularly those associated with profound immunosuppression, rashes remain prevalent, especially in those who do not have consistent HIV care. This review focuses on rashes almost exclusively related to HIV and rashes that have unusual presentations because of HIV infection.

INFECTIONS
Acute HIV Exanthem

Although it is difficult to recognize a patient with acute retroviral syndrome, emergency physicians are the most likely to encounter these patients. This syndrome is estimated to occur in one-half to two-thirds of persons infected with HIV, but is often misdiagnosed as a viral syndrome or infectious mononucleosis.[2] The symptom complex can include fever, malaise, myalgias, pharyngitis, lymphadenopathy, headache or other central nervous system abnormalities (photophobia, encephalitis, or meningitis), and rash in 30% to 50% of patients.[3–5] The rash is usually a maculopapular or macular eruption on the face, trunk, and upper extremities. Inclusion of the palms and soles can mimic secondary syphilis. Oral lesions are usually present, ranging from erythema to ulcers, which can cause severe dysphagia. Laboratory abnormalities can include leukopenia and thrombocytopenia. HIV antibody tests, whether serum- or oral fluid-based, will usually be negative acutely, and can take several months to seroconvert. Although not feasible to check in the emergency department (ED), viral loads will often be more than 1 million copies.

It is vital that the emergency physician consider acute retroviral syndrome in the differential diagnosis of acute viral infection in the appropriate host, and counsel the

[a] Division of Infectious Disease, University of Maryland School of Medicine, 29 South Greene Street, Suite 300, Baltimore, MD 21201, USA
[b] Department of Emergency Medicine, University of Maryland School of Medicine, 110 South Paca Street, 6th Floor, Suite 200, Baltimore, MD 21202, USA
* Corresponding author.
E-mail address: mkhambat@medicine.umaryland.edu

Emerg Med Clin N Am 28 (2010) 355–368
doi:10.1016/j.emc.2010.01.001
0733-8627/10/$ – see front matter © 2010 Elsevier Inc. All rights reserved.

emed.theclinics.com

patient to receive an HIV test as soon as possible. If not, HIV infection can remain undiagnosed for several years, as the symptom complex self-resolves in 1 to 3 weeks, and the patient does not seek further medical care.

Herpes Simplex Virus

In patients with HIV, herpes simplex virus (HSV) lesions occur more often, are more frequently atypical, and are less likely to self-resolve compared with patients not infected with HIV.[6] HSV is the most common viral infection in the patient infected with HIV, and as CD4 decreases to less than 100 cells/mm^3, the prevalence has been estimated to be as high as 27%.[7]

HSV lesions usually present as grouped vesicles on an erythematous base around the mouth, esophagus, genitals, perianal areas, and distal fingers. With advanced HIV immunodeficiency, the lesions can progress to persistent deep ulcers or coalesce and extend into mucosal and deep cutaneous layers. Necrosis, bleeding, and severe pain can occur, leading to an inability to eat or drink and requiring hospitalization for parental acyclovir (**Fig. 1**). If the patient can swallow, oral acyclovir compound drugs are usually effective. Valacyclovir has the highest oral bioavailability.

Varicella Zoster Virus

Herpes zoster (HZ) can be the initial presentation of a patient's immunodeficiency. HIV testing should be performed in those less than 65 years of age, who are not expected to have waning natural immunity. HZ affects 3% to 4% of patients infected with HIV.[8] The eruption is classically unidermatomal or multidermatomal, but with advanced HIV infection, can also present as disseminated disease.[9] HZ can be a recurrent event in 20% to 30% of patients with HIV.[10] Varicella zoster virus (VZV) can also cause severe primary chicken pox in an unexposed adult host.

With advanced HIV, VZV can present with atypical lesions. The most common are hyperkeratotic papules that do not follow a dermatomal pattern. The papules can persist for months to years. Another atypical manifestation is ecthymatous VZV, which appears as multiple ulcers of 1 to 3 cm with a central black eschars and a rim of vesicles.[11] Tzanck smears have a low yield. Direct immunofluorescence assay (DFA) and viral cultures are more sensitive, but a skin biopsy is required because there are no vesicles to provide a fluid sample. This is typically deferred to a dermatologist.

Zoster lesions, especially on the face, can be superinfected with *Streptococcus pyogenes* or *Staphylococcus aureus*, causing an impetigo-type lesion (**Fig. 2**). The

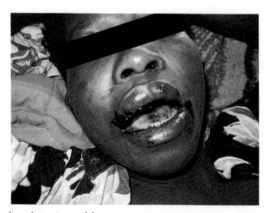

Fig. 1. Herpes simplex virus stomatitis.

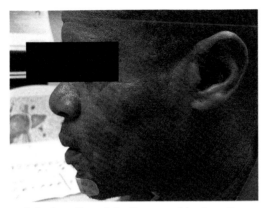

Fig. 2. Herpes zoster of the face. Superinfection resembles impetigo.

emergency medicine physician should treat the VZV infection and the secondary infection.

HZ can present without a rash in the immunocompromised host, and is known as zoster sine herpete.[12] Patients describe a deep-seated burning pain at the involved dermatome, and can present with complaints of chest pain, back pain, or abdominal pain. Patients may or may not have had zoster in the same dermatome in the past. The astute clinician will inquire whether the patient has ever had shingles, and if so, might elicit the helpful history that the pain "feels the same as my zoster." The lack of rash is not complete in many cases of zoster sine herpete, and a careful examination of the skin may reveal 1 or 2 vesicular or papular lesions.

The antiviral drugs used to treat HZ vary in bioavailability, efficacy, and cost. Acyclovir is the least expensive drug and has the lowest oral absorption at 10% to 15%. The dose is 800 mg 5 times a day. Famciclovir is available in generic form and dosed at 500 mg 2 times daily. Valacyclovir is not available generically, and is dosed at 1 g 3 times daily. All treatment regimens are given for at least 7 days. Large randomized trials show that acyclovir is inferior to valacyclovir and famciclovir in measurements of time to pain resolution and the incidence of postherpetic neuralgia. Famciclovir and valacyclovir are equal in efficacy and safety.[13,14]

Dermatophytosis

Cutaneous dermatophytosis is generally more atypical, extensive, and severe in the patient infected with HIV.[15] Dermatophytosis can manifest as tinea corporis, cruris, faciei, pedis, manuum, or unguium. Tinea corporis is usually caused by *Tricophyton rubrum*. Tinea corporis can present in acute or chronic forms. The acute form is classic ringworm, with sharply marginated erythematous, scaly macules, that are often multiple (**Fig. 3**). In the chronic form, lesions often coalesce into much larger hyperpigmented plaques (**Fig. 4**). Standard topical treatments will suffice for the acute form, but the extensive lesions associated with the chronic form should be treated with oral antifungals. Treatment consists of several weeks of terbinafine, fluconazole, ketoconazole, or itraconazole. If the patient is on ART, caution is warranted because ketoconazole and itraconazole can cause adverse drug interactions with protease inhibitors and non-nucleoside reverse transcriptase inhibitors.

Onychomycosis is more common in HIV infection. Any adult with fungal involvement of most toenails and especially the fingernails should be tested for HIV.

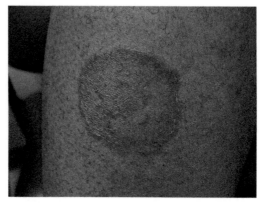

Fig. 3. Acute tinea corporis.

Tinea versicolor, also called pityriasis versicolor, is common and can be seen early in the course of HIV infection with CD4 counts more than 300 cells/mm^3.[8] It appears as sharply margined macules that can become confluent and cover an extensive area. The macules appear hypopigmented on dark skin, and hyperpigmented on light skin (**Fig. 5**). The macules have a fine scale that is better appreciated by scraping with a sharp-edged object. Microscopy of skin scrapings is diagnostic and reveals the yeast *Pitryrosporum ovale*, previously called *Malassezia furfur*, which also causes dandruff. The macules fluoresce green-yellow under a Wood lamp. Topical treatments such as selenium sulfide and ketoconazole cream can be used, but for widespread involvement and resistant cases, oral ketoconazole or itraconazole can be more convenient and effective. Because of possible interactions with ART medications and the lack of a well-established duration of treatment, candidates for oral therapy should be referred to their primary care or infectious disease provider.

Unusual Forms of Scabies

Scabies infection is the most common parasitic infection in patients with HIV.[16] The clinical presentation of scabies in the patient infected with HIV depends on their degree of immunosuppression. The typical presentation occurs in patients with relatively normal immune function. The fulminant, unusual, and more contagious forms

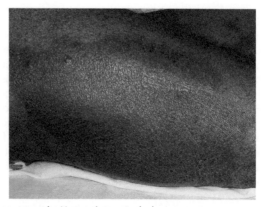

Fig. 4. Chronic tinea corporis. Hyperpigmented plaque.

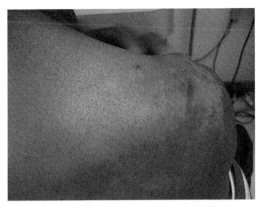

Fig. 5. Tinea versicolor. Lesions are hypopigmented on dark skin.

present with progressive immunosuppression. The 2 broad categories are exaggerated (also called papular or atypical) and crusted (also called hyperkeratotic or Norwegian). Patients can have both forms concurrently.[17]

Exaggerated scabies is highly pruritic and is characterized by generalized papules topped by a scabietic burrow (**Fig. 6**). Crusted scabies is less pruritic and presents as thick, white-gray plaques, which can be diffuse but are commonly localized to an area such as the extremities, scalp, face, back, or buttocks (**Fig. 7**). The plaques may not have typical burrows, but tend to form fissures, which may become secondarily infected.[17] Scrapings from the plaques will be laden with thousands to millions of mites, in contrast to scabies in immunocompetent hosts where no more than 5 or 10 mites are present.[18] Because of this high organism burden, patients with crusted scabies are extremely contagious and have been associated with institutional and health care-facility outbreaks, especially in the elderly. Treatment consists of topical permethrin 5% and oral ivermectin. Repeated weekly treatment courses are often required. There is no fixed length of treatment and skin scrapings to check for mites guide the duration of treatment.

Cryptococcosis

Primary dermal cryptococcosis is rare, and skin involvement usually indicates systemic disease. Skin lesions can have a variety of nonspecific presentations,

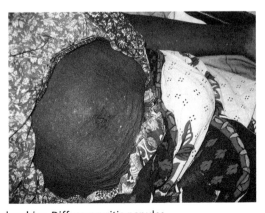

Fig. 6. Exaggerated scabies. Diffuse pruritic papules.

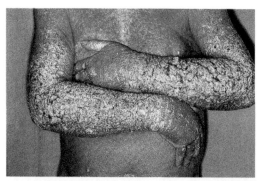

Fig. 7. Crusted scabies. Localized thick white-gray plaques. (*From* Mathieu ME, Wilson BB. Scabies. In: Mandell GL, Bennet JE, Dolin R, editors. Principles and practice of infectious diseases. 6th edition. Philadelphia: Elsevier; 2005. p. 3306; with permission.)

including papules, nodules, pustules, ulcers, and plaques (**Fig. 8**). Skin biopsy is needed to confirm the diagnosis. The treatment is the same as for systemic disease.

Histoplasmosis

Cutaneous histoplasmosis occurs in the setting of pulmonary or disseminated disease, as primary skin involvement is rare. The rash is nonspecific and appears as diffuse erythematous macules and papules, pustules, crusted ulcers, and psoriasiform papules. Diagnosis is made by skin biopsy, and treatment is the same as for systemic disease.

DRUG REACTIONS
Stevens-Johnson Syndrome and Toxic Epidermal Necrolysis

Patients with AIDS have up to 1000-fold higher risk of developing Stevens-Johnson syndrome (SJS) and toxic epidermal necrolysis (TEN) than the general population (**Fig. 9**).[19] Trimethoprim-sulfamethoxazole (TMP-SMX) is the most common cause of SJS and TEN in the patient infected with HIV because it is frequently prescribed for prophylaxis of pneumocystis pneumonia and toxoplasmosis, and treatment of methicillin-resistant staphylococcal aureus (MRSA) infections. The incidence of

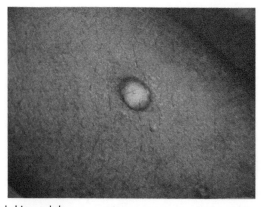

Fig. 8. Cryptococcal skin nodule.

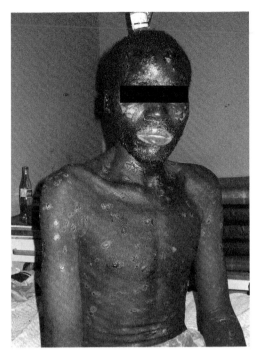

Fig. 9. Toxic epidermal necrolysis.

TMP-SMX-related TEN in AIDS patients is 980 per 1 million.[20] In comparison, the incidence of TEN, SJS or erythema multiforme in the general population taking TMP-SMX is 26 per 1 million.[21] Nevirapine is the antiretroviral most frequently associated with SJS/TEN, but other antiretrovirals can potentially cause SJS/TEN.

Treatment consists of discontinuing the offending agent, supportive care, hydration, minimizing adhesive tapes, which can cause additional sloughing, dermatology consult, and likely administration of intravenous high-dose immunoglobulin. Systemic antibiotics or transfer to a burn unit may also be indicated.

Sulfonamide-containing Medications

Allergies to sulfonamide-containing medications occur in about 1.5% to 3% of immunocompetent patients and up to 30% of patients infected with HIV.[22] The most common skin rash is a nonimmune-mediated generalized maculopapular or morbilliform exanthem (**Fig. 10**). The rash occurs within a few weeks of starting the drug, although the onset can occur months to years later. Lesions resolve rapidly after discontinuation of the offending agent, antihistamines and occasionally a short course of an oral steroid.

Rashes can also be immune-mediated. They may be urticarial and appear 1 to 3 days after starting the drug. Anaphylaxis can occur but is rare.

The sulfonamide hypersensitivity syndrome is an immune-mediated serum sickness that can occur 7 to 14 days after initiation of the drug. The syndrome includes fever and toxicity of 1 or more organs. Eosinophilia is sometimes present. The associated rash is lupuslike and can progress to SJS or TEN.[22] Treatment is supportive and includes withdrawal of the drug.

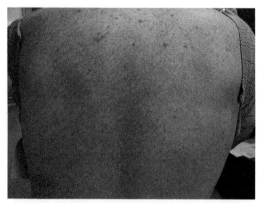

Fig. 10. Sulfa hypersensitivity. Diffuse erythematous maculopapular or morbilliform rash.

The most commonly prescribed sulfa is TMP-SMX. Desensitization is possible in more than 90% of patients who experience a mild rash to TMP-SMX. Several antiretrovirals have sulfa moieties as well, including atazanavir (Reyataz) and darunavir (Prezista), which usually cause mild rashes that do not require discontinuation of the drug.

ART-ASSOCIATED RASHES

Antiretroviral drugs can cause morbilliform eruptions. They are typically transient and are not associated with constitutional symptoms or laboratory abnormalities. They are treated with antihistamines. Discontinuation of ART is usually not necessary.

More serious rashes are associated with so-called hypersensitivity reactions. These are immune-related reactions that occur within a few weeks of initiating a drug. Nevirapine and abacavir are most commonly associated with hypersensitivity reactions, although other antiretrovirals have been implicated. The presentation mimics a nonspecific viral illness, with fever, malaise, and variable gastrointestinal and respiratory symptoms. Severe organ toxicity can occur, including myocarditis, hepatitis, and interstitial nephritis.[23] The rash is often subtle, resembling a mild nonspecific viral exanthem or appearing urticarial. Laboratory abnormalities are nonspecific and non-diagnostic, including leukopenia, anemia, thrombocytopenia, and increased levels of creatinine and liver enzymes.

The duty of the emergency physician is to include hypersensitivity reactions in the differential diagnosis of the patient infected with HIV who recently started ART and presents with an apparent viral illness. Discontinuation of the drug will resolve the reaction, whereas continuation of the offending drug can lead to worsening symptoms and organ toxicity that will require hospitalization. Corticosteroid and antihistamine medications do not generally hasten the resolution of the reaction. Communicating a suspicion of hypersensitivity reaction to the patient's primary care/HIV physician is essential to successful management.

Unique rashes associated with specific antiretrovirals are discussed in the following sections.

Zidovudine (AZT, Retrovir, Zidovir, Contained in Combivir, Trizivir)

Melanonychia or longitudinal, darkly pigmented nail bands have been noted in about 50% of patients taking a drug containing zidovudine (including Combivir and Trizivir) (**Fig. 11**). This is more common in dark-skinned individuals and is caused by the deposition of melanin. This condition may or may not reverse after discontinuation of the

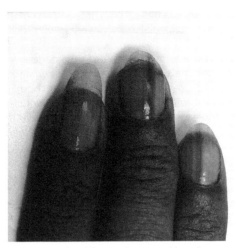

Fig. 11. Melanonychia. Longitudinal hyperpigmented bands.

drug. Zidovudine can also cause hyperpigmentation of the skin and oral mucosa, which is usually reversible.[24]

Nevirapine (Viramune)

A maculopapular erythematous eruption occurs in 16% of adults within the 6 weeks of starting nevirapine.[25] If a patient experiences this rash within the first 18 weeks of starting nevirapine, transaminase levels should be checked. If they are more than 5 times the upper limit of normal, nevirapine should be discontinued.

Severe rashes occur in up to 1% of patients taking nevirapine. These include SJS, TEN, and severe hypersensitivity reactions. Organ failure, including hepatic failure, has been reported.[26,27]

Atazanavir (Reyataz, Latazanavir, Zrivada)

Scleral icterus and jaundice occur in 7% to 8% of patients taking atazanavir.[28] Atazanavir causes a dose-related reversible inhibition of UDP-glucuronosyl transferase, which leads to increased levels of indirect bilirubin. If the increases are mild, and the patient is otherwise asymptomatic, the drug can be continued. Indications for discontinuing the drug include persistent itching from high levels of bilirubin or patient choice for cosmetic reasons. Transaminase increases do not occur as a result of atazanavir, and other causes should be considered if transaminase abnormalities are present.

Enfuvirtide (T-20, Fuzeon)

Enfuvirtide is injected subcutaneously, and most patients develop an injection site reaction including pruritus, erythema, induration, ecchymosis, nodules, and cysts. Reactions may be at multiple sites and last for up to a week. Occasionally, the injection site can develop cellulitis or abscess.

OTHER RASHES
Psoriasis

Psoriasis affects 1% to 2% of the general population, but affects 1.3% to 5% of patients infected with HIV.[8] As psoriasis can be the first presentation of HIV infection,

HIV testing should be considered in a patient who has worsening of stable psoriasis or develops psoriasis de novo, especially in patients with risk factors for HIV infection.[29,30]

The severity of the presentation often correlates to the degree of immune suppression.[31] Psoriasis vulgaris, classically appearing with thick white scale, may present with widespread involvement covering almost the entire body surface (**Fig. 12**). Pustular psoriasis may develop, with multiple sterile pustules within erythematous plaques. The pustules may coalesce into large bullae of pus. Another severe form is erythrodermic psoriasis, characterized by a full-body, erythematous rash that exfoliates.

The management of psoriasis in patients infected with HIV is complicated by the need to avoid the typical immunosuppressive treatments used for psoriasis. Antiretroviral treatment itself can ameliorate lesions. Emergency department management should focus on recognizing the disease, evaluating for superinfection, and arranging follow-up with dermatology and infectious disease.

Seborrheic Dermatitis

Seborrheic dermatitis is 1 of the most common rashes seen in patients infected with HIV, affecting 85% of all patients at some point in their disease course.[32] Seborrheic dermatitis is seen at all stages of HIV infection, although advanced HIV immunosuppression correlates with more severe presentations. An adult with extensive seborrheic dermatitis should be tested for HIV if their status is not already known.

The causative organism is the yeast *Pitryrosproum ovale*, which also causes dandruff. The rash appears as yellow-white, sometimes greasy scales on hypopigmented and/or erythematous patches. In mild cases, seborrheic dermatitis appears on the face, particularly around the nose and eyebrows, the scalp, and upper chest (**Fig. 13**). In more severe cases, the back, axillae, and groin can be involved. Treatment is topical antifungals such as miconazole or ketoconazole. If the rash is inflamed and erythematous, topical medium potency steroids can also be used. Seborrheic dermatitis typically improves with ART.

Pruritic Papular Eruption and Eosinophilic Folliculitis

Pruritic papular eruption (PPE) is one of the most common causes of pruritus in patients infected with HIV. The prevalence is 11% to 46%, with the lowest in North

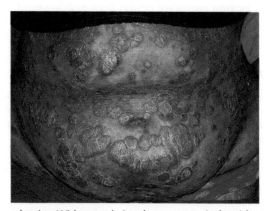

Fig. 12. Psoriasis vulgaris. Widespread involvement typical with advanced immune suppression.

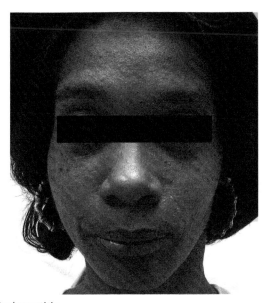

Fig. 13. Seborrheic dermatitis.

America and Europe and highest in Africa and Southeast Asia.[33] PPE is a marker for advanced HIV, appearing predominately when the CD4 count is less than 100 cells/mm^3.[32]

PPE appears as multiple papules, typically symmetric, on the face, trunk, and extensor surfaces of the extremities with sparing of the palms and soles. Because of the chronic nature of PPE, the papules are often excoriated and develop inflammation, hyperpigmentation, and scarring. Over time, severe inflammation causes the papules to become nodular in appearance (**Fig. 14**). The cause of PPE is unknown and there is no consensus on treatment. The pruritus is resistant to antihistamine antipruritics, but may improve with ART, warranting close follow-up with an infectious disease specialist.

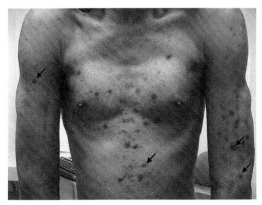

Fig. 14. Pruritic papular eruption. Nodules develop because of chronic inflammation (*arrows*).

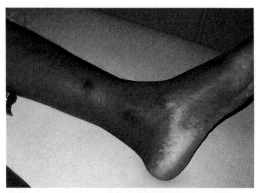

Fig. 15. Kaposi sarcoma.

Eosinophilic folliculitis (EF) is closely related to and easily confused with PPE. Histology studies are sometimes needed to distinguish between them. EF is commonly seen when the CD4 count is less than 300 cells/mm^3.[34] Like PPE, EF presents with pruritic papules, but the distribution is typically confined to the face, neck, upper arms, and torso above the nipple line. Infrequent sterile pustules also distinguish EF from PPE. As its name suggests, EF is associated with eosinophilia, as is PPE, and eosinophilic infiltrates around affected follicles on histology studies. The cause of EF is unknown. The diagnosis is made clinically. Treatment includes ultraviolet-B light therapy and topical steroids, and should be initiated by a dermatologist or infectious disease specialist.

Patients can develop EF or complain of worsening EF during immune reconstitution inflammatory syndrome.[34] Patients should be informed that it is an expected result of ART, and with continuation of the HIV medication, it should resolve in the next few months.

Kaposi Sarcoma

Kaposi sarcoma (KS) is a vascular neoplasm that affects visceral organs as well as mucocutaneous surfaces. KS is an AIDS-defining illness and generally indicates advanced HIV. The skin lesions are violaceous macules, nodules, patches, or plaques (**Fig. 15**). The lesions can grow and coalesce. They are often asymptomatic, but can ulcerate and become secondarily infected. KS is treated with a combination of chemotherapy and ART, but ART alone has led to remission in isolated cutaneous KS.[32]

ACKNOWLEDGMENTS

The authors wish to thank Neha Umesh Sheth, PharmD for her valuable input and research on drug reactions.

REFERENCES

1. Coopman SA, Johnson RA, Platt R, et al. Cutaneous disease and drug reactions in HIV infection. N Engl J Med 1993;328:1670–4.
2. Weismann K, Petersen CS, Sondergaard J, et al. Skin signs in AIDS: textbook of AIDS/HIV infection-related dermatology. Copenhagen (Denmark): Munksgaard; 1998.

3. Brehmer-Anderson E, Torssander J. The exanthema of acute (primary) HIV infection: identification of a characteristic histopathologic picture? Acta Derm Venereol 1990;70:85–7.
4. Hulsebosch HJ, Claessen FA, VanGinkel CJ, et al. Human immunodeficiency virus examthen. J Am Acad Dermatol 1990;23:483–6.
5. Abrams DI. Clinical manifestations of HIV infection, including persistent generalized lymphadenopathy and AIDS-related complex. J Am Acad Dermatol 1990;22:1217–22.
6. Severson JL, Tyring SK. Relation between herpes simplex viruses and human immunodeficiency infections. Arch Dermatol 1999;135:1393–7.
7. Goodman DS, Teplitz ED, Wishner A, et al. Prevalence of cutaneous disease in patient with acquired immunodeficiency syndrome (AIDS) or AIDS-related complex. J Am Acad Dermatol 1987;17:210–20.
8. Zalla MJ, Daniel WP, Fransway AF. Dermatologic manifestations of human immunodeficiency virus infection. Mayo Clin Proc 1992;67:1089–108.
9. Cohen PR, Beltrani VP, Grossman ME. Disseminated herpes zoster in patients with human immunodeficiency virus infection. Am J Med 1988;84:1076–80.
10. Perronne C, Lazanas M, Leport C, et al. Varicella in patients infected with the human immunodeficiency virus. Arch Dermatol 1990;126:1033–6.
11. Gnann JW. Varicella-zoster virus: atypical presentations and unusual complications. J Infect Dis 2002;186(Suppl 1):S91–8.
12. Gilden DH, Wright RR, Schneck SA, et al. Zoster sine herpete, a clinical variant. Ann Neurol 1994;35(5):530–3.
13. Beutner KR, Friedman DJ, Forzpaniak C, et al. Valacyclovir compared to acyclovir for the improved therapy for herpes zoster in immunocompetent adults. Antimicrobial Agents Chemother 1995;39:1546–53.
14. Tyring SK, Beutner KR, Tucker BA, et al. Antiviral therapy for herpes zoster: randomized, controlled clinical trial of valacyclovir and famciclovir therapy in immunocompetent patients 50 years and older. Arch Fam Med 2000;9(9):863–9.
15. Burkhart CN, Chang H, Gotwald L. Tinea corporis in human immunodeficiency virus-positive patient: case report and assessment of oral therapy. Int J Dermatol 2003;42:839–43.
16. Castano-Molina C, Cockerell CJ. Diagnosis and treatment of infectious diseases in HIV-infected hosts. Dermatol Clin 1997;15:267–83.
17. Thappa DM, Karthikeyan K. Exaggerated scabies: a marker for HIV infection. Indian Pediatr 2002;39:875–6.
18. Mathieu ME, Wilson BB. Scabies. In: Mandell GL, Bennet JE, Dolin R, editors. Principles and practice of infectious diseases. 6th edition. Philadelphia: Elsevier; 2005. p. 3304–7.
19. Rzanky B, Hamouda O, Schoph E. Incidence of Stevens-Johnson syndrome, and toxic epidermal necrolysis in patients with acquired immunodeficiency syndrome in Germany. Arch Dermatol 1993;129:1059.
20. Saiag P, Caumes E, Chosidow O, et al. Drug-induced toxic epidermal necrolysis in patients infected with human immunodeficiency virus. J Am Acad Dermatol 1992;26:567–74.
21. Chan HL, Stern RS, Arndt KA, et al. The incidence of erythema multiforme, Stevens-Johnson syndrome and toxic epidermal necrolysis; a population based study with particular reference to reactions caused by drugs among outpatients. Arch Dermatol 1990;126:43–7.

22. Brackett CC, Singh H, Block JH. Likelihood and mechanisms of cross-allergenicity between sulfonamide antibiotics and other drugs containing a sulfonamide functional group. Pharmacotherapy 2004;24(7):856–70.

23. Anderson JA, Adkinson NF. Allergic reactions to drugs and biologic agents. JAMA 1987;258:2891–9.

24. Kong HH, Myers SA. Cutaneous effects of highly active antiretroviral therapy in HIV-infected patients. Dermatol Ther 2005;18:58–66.

25. Pollard RB, Robinson P, Dransfield K. Safety profile of nevirapine, a non-nucleoside reverse transcriptase inhibitor for the treatment of human immunodeficiency virus infection. Clin Ther 1998;20:1071–92.

26. Warren KJ, Boxwell DE, Kim NY, et al. Nevirapine-associated Stevens-Johnson syndrome. Lancet 1998;351:567.

27. Barner A, Myers M. Nevirapine and rashes. Lancet 1998;351:1133.

28. LeTiec C, Barrail A, Goujard C, et al. Clinical pharmacokinetics and summary of efficacy and tolerability of atazanavir. Clin Pharmacokinet 2005;44(10):1035–50.

29. Goodman DS, Teplitz ED, Wisher A, et al. Prevalence of cutaneous disease in patients with acquired immunodeficiency syndrome. J Am Acad Dermatol 1986;17:210–20.

30. Johnson TM, Duvic M, Rapini RP, et al. AIDS exacerbates psoriasis. N Engl J Med 1985;313:1415.

31. Obuch ML, Maurer TA, Becker B, et al. Psoriasis and human immunodeficiency virus infection. J Am Acad Dermatol 1992;275:667–73.

32. Rigopoulos J, Paparizos V, Katsambas A. Cutaneous markers of HIV infection. Clin Dermatol 2004;22:487–98.

33. Eisman S. Pruritic papular eruptions of HIV-1. Dermatol Clin 2006;24:449–57.

34. Rajendran PM, Dolev JC, Heaphy MR, et al. Eosinophilic folliculitis: before and after the introduction of antiretroviral therapy. Arch Dermatol 2005;141:1227–31.

Rapid HIV Screening in the Emergency Department

Mercedes Torres, MD

KEYWORDS

- Human immunodeficiency virus • Emergency department
- Screening • Testing • Rapid • Diagnosis

In 2001 and then again in 2006, the Centers for Disease Control and Prevention (CDC) published guidelines recommending universal HIV screening in most outpatient and acute care settings, including emergency departments (EDs).[1] Since this recommendation was released, ED administrators have struggled to determine feasible methods for offering HIV screening in their EDs. This has proven to be a significant challenge considering recent trends in ED care, including overcrowding and increasing numbers of boarded patients. According to the CDC, all outpatient and acute care settings in communities with a prevalence of HIV infection greater than 1% should be equipped to offer universal HIV screening. The goal is to improve the overall public health of Americans by detecting HIV infection before the development of symptoms using reliable, inexpensive screening tests, and initiate disease-modifying treatment, therefore decreasing morbidity and mortality from the disease. An additional goal is to prevent the spread of HIV by detecting infected patients sooner and providing counseling regarding prevention strategies.[1]

In theory, the ED is the ideal location for this type of universal screening program. The ED is the primary point of care for numerous patients without access to health care, including those at highest risk for contracting HIV. When a traditional sexually transmitted disease (STD) clinic HIV screening program was compared with an ED-based HIV screening program, the ED program showed a measurable advantage, as 30% more new infections were detected. This improvement was accomplished with only a fraction of the number of tests performed in the STD clinic (10%) and fewer dedicated staff, further demonstrating the diagnostic power of an ED-based screening program.[2]

Although the public health benefits of universal HIV screening are significant, the practicality of such a policy is not as clear. As one 2008 survey demonstrated, only 50% of academic EDs had rapid HIV testing within their department, and half of these

Department of Emergency Medicine, University of Maryland School of Medicine, 101 South Paca Street, Sixth Floor, Suite 200, Baltimore, MD 21202, USA
E-mail address: mercedet@gmail.com

Emerg Med Clin N Am 28 (2010) 369–380
doi:10.1016/j.emc.2010.01.008
0733-8627/10/$ – see front matter © 2010 Elsevier Inc. All rights reserved.

EDs restricted its use to occupational exposures.[3] This survey further showed that slightly more than half of responding EDs had the ability to link patients to care after an HIV diagnosis, and only 13% had developed a policy regarding the routine screening of patients for HIV.[3] Importantly, the survey was distributed to academic EDs, which often maintain greater resources and larger staffing levels as compared with most community EDs in the country. In addition, academic EDs are often more capable of obtaining grants or supplemental funding for these types of public health initiatives. Even with those distinct advantages, implementation of the CDC guidelines has been fraught with difficulties, as shown by the low numbers of respondents with any resources or programs for HIV testing in this survey.[3]

To address some of the difficulties associated with implementing a universal HIV screening program in an ED, the CDC revised the initial guidelines released in 2001 with the following changes[1]:

- HIV screening is recommended for all patients once notified that they will be screened unless the patient explicitly declines the test ("opt-out" screening)
- Separate written informed consent for HIV testing should not be required; general consent for medical care should be considered sufficient to encompass consent for HIV testing
- Prevention counseling should not be required with HIV screening or diagnostic testing programs.

These revisions acknowledge some of the unique difficulties of conducting a universal screening program within an acute care setting, such as the ED. As this article explores, there are still many hurdles to developing a successful, sustainable ED-based universal HIV screening program.

TYPES OF HIV TESTS

There are several commercially available Food and Drug Administration (FDA)-approved rapid HIV tests. Although conventional HIV tests are available and used in many settings, they are not ideal for use in the ED, as they cannot provide same-day preliminary results and they typically require a higher level of laboratory expertise and time to perform. The development of rapid HIV tests has paved the way for HIV screening in a multitude of settings, including the ED. FDA-approved rapid HIV tests include those run on oral fluid, whole blood, or serum/plasma, as shown in **Table 1**. All tests run on whole blood or oral fluids are Clinical Laboratory Improvement Amendments (CLIA)-waived, indicating that there are less intensive laboratory procedural and training requirements. Recommendations are that positive rapid test results are reported as preliminary until confirmatory testing is performed.[4,5]

Each of the tests listed in **Table 1** has unique features that make it more or less desirable depending on the specific resources of a particular ED. The OraQuick Advance HIV-1/2, manufactured by Orasure Technologies Inc (Bethlehem, PA, USA), requires a 5-μL specimen volume and can be run on oral fluid, whole blood, or serum/plasma. This test is the only one with the option of oral fluid, decreasing the equipment required to obtain samples as well as the risk to the person obtaining the sample for testing. The read time is 20 to 40 minutes and the shelf life is approximately 6 months. The test is approved to detect both HIV-1 and -2. The UniGold Recombigen HIV is only approved for detection of HIV-1. This test can be run on whole blood or plasma/serum, and requires a 40-μL specimen volume. Results are available in 10 to 20 minutes and the shelf life is 1 year. Similar to the UniGold Recombigen test, Clearview Complete HIV-1/2 can be run on whole blood or plasma/serum, and

Table 1		
FDA-approved rapid HIV test types, sensitivities, and specificities		
Oral Fluid	Sensitivity (95% CI)	Specificity (95% CI)
OraQuick Advance HIV-1/2	99.3 (98.4–99.7)	99.8 (99.6–99.9)
Whole blood		
OraQuick Advance HIV-1/2	99.6 (98.5–99.9)	100 (99.7–100)
UniGold Recombigen HIV	100 (99.5–100)	99.7 (99.0–100
Clearview HIV-1/2 Stat-Pak	99.7 (98.9–100)	99.9 (98.6–100)
Clearview Complete HIV-1/2	99.7 (98.9–100)	99.9 (98.6–100)
Serum/Plasma		
OraQuick Advance HIV-1/2	99.6 (98.9–99.8)	99.9 (99.6–99.9)
UniGold Recombigen HIV	100 (99.5–100)	99.8 (99.3–100)
Clearview HIV-1/2 Stat-Pak	99.7 (98.9–100)	99.9 (98.6–100)
Clearview Complete HIV-1/2	99.7 (98.9–100)	99.9 (98.6–100)
Reveal G3 HIV-1	99.8 (99.2–100)	99.1 (98.9–99.4)
Multispot HIV-1/HIV-2	100 (99.9–100)	99.9 (99.8–100)

Data from Centers for Disease Control and Prevention (CDC). FDA-approved rapid HIV antibody screening tests. Available at: http://www.cdc.gov/hiv/topics/testing/rapid/rt-comparison.htm. Accessed August 2, 2009.

requires a 2.5-μL specimen volume, the smallest of all available rapid tests. This test is read in 15 to 20 minutes and its shelf life is 2 years. The Clearview Stat-Pak HIV-1/2 is similar to the Clearview Complete test with regard to the aforementioned characteristics, with the exception of the required specimen volume of 5 μL.[4,5]

The Reveal G3 HIV-1 and Multispot HIV-1/HIV-2 are both categorized as moderate complexity under CLIA, as they both can only be run on plasma/serum. Reveal G3 is only approved for HIV-1 and requires a 2-step process by laboratory technicians on a 40-μL specimen volume, but results are immediate (within 5 minutes). The shelf-life is 2 years. The Multispot test distinguishes HIV-1 from HIV-2. This test requires a 30-μL specimen volume, but involves several timed reagent and wash steps. Its shelf life is 3 months at room temperature and 1 year in the refrigerator.[4,5]

UNIVERSAL HIV SCREENING VERSUS TARGETED HIV TESTING

According to the 2006 CDC recommendations, patients in acute care settings with a prevalence of HIV greater than 1% should be offered screening in a nontargeted fashion. The goal of this strategy is to diagnose asymptomatic HIV-infected patients who present to the ED for unrelated complaints. Targeted testing strategies identify specific groups of patients with identified risk factors for HIV, while universal screening aims to test as many patients as possible regardless of their complaint or risk profile. This strategy is aimed at identifying the 24% to 27% of HIV-infected patients who are not aware of their status.[2,6] Multiple studies have been conducted to determine the value of universal screening as compared with targeted testing for ED patients. Although the benefit of identifying patients at earlier stages of HIV by screening all patients is clear, the effectiveness of this strategy has not been established.

In a recently published study from Highland Hospital in Oakland, California, researchers concurrently collected data regarding patients screened for HIV as compared with patients whose providers had a clinical suspicion for HIV and therefore initiated HIV testing as part of their diagnostic evaluation. The results demonstrated that 0.7% of almost 8000 patients screened for HIV were confirmed positive, while 3% of 1500 who were targeted for testing by providers were positive. Although the yield of targeted screening was clearly higher, the severity of disease for those diagnosed with targeted testing was greater. Sixty percent of the HIV-positive patients who were targeted for testing had CD4 counts less than 200, as compared with 28% of those identified with screening. Further analysis of the results examined the rate of identification of HIV-positive patients among only those admitted to the hospital. The researchers demonstrated that 59% of those diagnosed with HIV through their ED-based testing would have been missed in this case. Analysis of the data based on demographics attempting to identify a target group of patients to be tested showed that testing male, non-Hispanic patients between the ages of 34 and 54 years would have identified a majority of the patients who ultimately tested positive. However, this analysis also revealed that prevalence remained greater than 0.1% in every major demographic group, therefore justifying screening of all groups as per CDC recommendations.[7]

Several other studies have demonstrated similar results, weighing the benefit of early identification under a universal screening protocol against the greater efficiency of targeted testing. From January 2003 until April 2004, ED staff at Cook County Hospital offered both HIV screening and provider-initiated HIV testing. A significantly greater proportion of patients who were referred for HIV testing by their provider tested positive (11.6% vs 1.2%). Of these patients, the provider-referred patients had a greater proportion of patients with initial CD4 counts less than 200 (82% vs 45%). Of note, more than half of HIV positives in each group did not have a history of any known risk factors. The investigators estimated that 42% of new HIV diagnoses would have been missed if testing was only offered to those considered at risk. Their conclusion emphasizes that targeted, risk-based testing is not an effective strategy for identifying patients early in the course of HIV infection, as many patients do not perceive or disclose their risks to health care providers.[2]

One key problem with risk-based screening is that many patients who are ultimately diagnosed with HIV do not perceive themselves to be at risk. When patients have declined HIV screening and have been asked the reasons for this, they frequently note that they do not consider themselves to be at risk for contracting HIV. In one survey, among the reasons cited by patients refusing HIV testing, 60% noted no perceived risk for HIV, 16% reported a recent negative test, and 15% stated that they did not have time to do the test during their ED visit. The fear and stigma which once characterized public rejection of HIV testing programs have now been replaced with false perceptions of personal risk for HIV.[8,9] Public awareness that traditional risk factors for HIV, such as men who have sex with men or a history of intravenous drug use (IVDU), account for fewer and fewer new HIV infections each year has lagged the reality of the situation. In some high-prevalence settings, up to 25% of new HIV infections are found in patients with no clear risk factor.[10] As such, it appears difficult to design a "target" group for HIV testing that would encompass the majority of undiagnosed HIV infected patients in any given population.

In addition to patient's not perceiving their own risk of HIV infection, research has demonstrated that many health care providers are equally bad at identifying patients at risk for HIV. In a retrospective study of 348 patients diagnosed with HIV, 34% were found to have had at least one clinical encounter during the 3 years before diagnosis. Only 9 of those 120 patients with previous encounters had an HIV test performed. The median number of visits per patient before HIV diagnosis was 2, with 58% treated in an urgent care center, 50% treated in an ED, 29% treated in a primary care clinic, and

16% having been admitted. Even at the time of diagnosis, ED or urgent care center providers identified only 10% of the 120 patients who were found to be HIV-infected. When the diagnoses of these patients during previous encounters were analyzed, there was no indication of the presence of increased risk of HIV. However, investigators note that on interview after HIV diagnosis, 75% of these newly diagnosed patients did identify a more traditional risk factor. These data point to 2 shortcomings of targeted screening programs. First, emergency physicians are less likely to have the time to elucidate a history of risk for HIV during their brief encounter with a patient with whom they have no established relationship. Second, most risk-based targeted testing identifies patients at risk based on their chief complaint, which is often unrelated to their risk profile for HIV infection. Given these constraints of targeted testing and the delays associated with diagnosis in targeted testing programs, the authors of this study argue for universal HIV screening in acute care settings.[11]

In summary, the debate regarding the value of universal HIV screening compared with risk-based HIV testing in acute care settings focuses on multiple complex issues. As many studies have demonstrated, although risk-based testing provides a higher yield on HIV testing efforts, it misses many patients who do not have, or are unwilling to disclose, traditional risk factors and may be earlier in the stage of their HIV infection. These are precisely those patients that public health officials are trying to identify to initiate early treatment, while also protecting others to whom they may unknowingly transmit the virus. While it would be much more efficient to target populations for HIV testing, the value of these efficiencies has been called into question amid the realization that determining a target group is not a straightforward task and will invariably miss many nontraditional positives.[6,11]

OPT-IN VERSUS OPT-OUT CONSENT FOR TESTING

Obtaining consent for HIV testing has traditionally been a time-consuming process. Most providers were mandated by hospital policies and state-based guidelines to provide separate HIV testing consent forms with specific pretest information regarding risk factors for HIV, prevention strategies, and the HIV test itself. When initial CDC recommendations regarding HIV screening in acute care settings were developed in 2001, they were based on an opt-in strategy of offering testing to patients and only performing it after the patient agreed to the test with a separate consent form. In 2006, this strategy was revised after many pilot programs demonstrated that the time and energy required in the consent process was hindering the ability to perform a maximal number of tests. The new strategy, known as opt-out testing, involves notifying each patient that they will be tested for HIV during their ED visit unless they specifically decline the test. In addition, the informed consent requirements have been loosened, eliminating the required separate consent and encompassing consent for an HIV test into the general consent for medical care in the ED.[1]

Opt-out HIV testing has become the recommendation in an effort to increase the number of ED patients screened for HIV. As projects in overcrowded urban EDs in Los Angeles and New York have demonstrated, the use of a lengthy separate consent form with an opt-in strategy for recruiting patients results in a low yield of HIV tests offered (2%–4% of total ED visits). This result differs from that of a modified approach attempted in an Oakland, California ED, where opt-in consent was still used, but consent was truncated to an 11-line script reviewed at the time of triage by the nurse rather than during a separate meeting with an HIV counselor. This modification, although still employing an opt-in strategy, allowed HIV testing to be offered to a greater proportion of ED patients (47.7%). Debate regarding the value of truncated consent exists, as a much smaller proportion of patients offered screening actually accepted the testing in Oakland (52%) than in New York (84%) and Los Angeles (98.3%). The opt-out strategy is offered as a more streamlined approach to consent and testing for all of these programs.[7,12]

In another study to measure patient acceptance of opt-in HIV testing, almost 2100 patients were offered rapid HIV testing using this strategy, with only 31.9% accepting the test. Patients rejecting the test often cited a lack of perceived risk for HIV or concern for their primary medical complaint as reasons for deferring HIV testing.[9] The authors of this study and of others with similar results point to opt-out testing as a way to possibly increase acceptance rates of testing by making the HIV test a routine part of the medical encounter, rather than an added service, available based on a patient's desire or perceived need for that service.[9,11,13] This has been demonstrated at STD and prenatal clinics, where opt-out screening has increased rates and acceptance of HIV screening.[1]

In an attempt to gauge public acceptance of an opt-out versus opt-in strategy for consent for HIV screening in the ED, researchers in Denver performed a cross-sectional survey of ED patients. Of the 529 patients interviewed for this survey, equal numbers of patients (81%) expressed a willingness to be tested for HIV in a nontargeted opt-out versus a nontargeted opt-in HIV screening program. The highest rate of acceptance of HIV testing in the surveyed group remained associated with physician referral for the test (93%). In addition, surveyed patients were asked if consent for HIV should be separate from the general consent for medical care. Fifty percent felt that the consent should remain separate, demonstrating a much lower level of acceptance of this aspect of the CDC recommendations.[14]

PRACTICAL APPROACHES TO PRE- AND POSTTEST COUNSELING IN THE ED

One of the largest obstacles to implementing HIV testing in an ED is ensuring that pre- and posttest counseling are available for all patients. In the past, this type of counseling required lengthy discussions with patients to gauge their understanding of their risk factors, discuss prevention strategies, explain the testing procedure, and address specific concerns related to each patient's particular circumstance.[10] Although extensive counseling is clearly beneficial to many patients, dispelling myths about HIV, teaching important prevention strategies, and addressing their concerns, it has proven burdensome to ED staff who are already operating in a setting of inadequate staffing and overcrowding. As such, the CDC recognized this barrier to the effective implementation of an HIV screening program and has revised its recommendations regarding pre- and posttest counseling. The current recommendation highlights the importance of providing oral or written information to all patients screened regarding the meaning of positive and negative test results and a description of HIV infection. It is recommended that written information about HIV be available in multiple languages and that patients are given an opportunity to ask questions about any of this prior to testing. Specifically noted in the recommendations, prevention counseling should not be required as part of the screening program but rather as a community outreach activity aside from screening.[1]

Removal of portions of the previously offered HIV pretest counseling has been met with some resistance from professionals providing services to HIV patients, who have emphasized the importance of tailoring counseling to meet each specific patient's needs and the inability to do so with the abbreviated pretest education suggested.[15] To measure public acceptance of an abbreviated or absent pretest education session during HIV screening, 529 patients presenting to a Denver ED were asked if they felt that counseling was necessary before or after HIV testing. Only 34% indicated that they felt that it was needed in either of these circumstances.[14]

While these recommendations have abbreviated the time-consuming job of pretest counseling in ED-based screening programs, some pretest counseling is still typically performed. In EDs with available staff, dedicated HIV counselors or social workers are often assigned this task. Unfortunately, due to financial and staffing constraints, this is not the case for most EDs. As a result, ED administrators have piloted programs that combine video-based pretest counseling with written material and a brief question/answer opportunity to meet the pretest counseling needs of screened ED patients. A randomized, controlled noninferiority trial was performed in one ED considering the implementation of video-based pretest counseling to assess its ability to communicate the appropriate information as compared with face-to-face discussion. The 9.5-minute video used focused on the definition of HIV, nature of the disease, transmission, HIV testing process, interpretation of test results, and prevention. Participants were randomly assigned to video or in-person pretest education and then given a questionnaire to assess their understanding of several key concepts relayed in both sessions. There was no significant difference found in the scores of patients receiving pretest education from a counselor versus a video. There were significant differences in scores based on level of education, but not type of pretest counseling.[16]

Similar results were found in another randomized controlled trial of standard in-person pretest counseling versus video-based pretest counseling in an inner city ED a few years earlier. This study used a 10-question measure of retained information for both groups, which was at a fifth grade reading level and available in English and Spanish. Ninety-one percent of interviewed patients felt that the video provided sufficient information for them to provide consent for testing and 98% ultimately ended up consenting to testing. Similar levels of retention of information were measured for both groups. The investigators identified multiple advantages to video-based pretest counseling, including the increased accessibility for patients with limited literacy, the consistency of information provided in multiple languages, the cost-effectiveness, the ability to fill time patients spend waiting in the ED, and the availability at all hours. Shortcomings of video-based education include the lack of personal interaction, and the continued requirement for someone to solicit and answer any questions patients may have after viewing the video.[17]

Video has also been proposed as a means of communicating posttest counseling information to screened patients. The cost-effectiveness of video as a posttest prevention counseling strategy was measured in a recent unmasked randomized trial. A 15-minute posttest counseling video geared to an eighth-grade reading level, available in English and Spanish, focused on prevention strategies, including condom use and dental dams, interpretation of HIV results, partner notification, and issues of domestic violence. A true/false test was administered to 67 patients receiving traditional in-person posttest counseling and 61 patients receiving video-based posttest counseling. The results demonstrated that patients who viewed the video scored higher on the assessment than did those receiving in-person counseling, but within the margin of error. As such, both methods were determined to be equivalent based on scores on this test.[18]

Video-based education provided to patients screened for HIV has been characterized as impersonal and inadequate by HIV providers and counselors. In direct response to one of the previously referenced studies, HIV providers from Denver Health Sciences published an editorial acknowledging the usefulness of video in the ED setting, while emphasizing that it is not equivalent to or a substitution for in-person counseling. A clear distinction is made between video-based dissemination of information related to HIV and the personalized discussion of a counseling session. The investigators emphasize the importance of tailoring the counseling session to the specific circumstances presented by each individual patient, and highlight that this is impossible using a video.[15] These concerns must be weighed against the increasing pressure from the CDC to implement universal screening in the ED, where staff is limited, time is precious, and resources are slim.

In all studies reviewed, specific HIV results have been communicated to patients in person by a health care provider. In an effort to conserve the limited physician time available for education and counseling, many screening programs have nurses relay negative results to screened patients, while physicians or HIV counselors typically inform patients of positive results.[7] Another idea proposed for streamlining the pre- and posttest counseling components of HIV screening in the ED, especially during off-hours when additional staff is not available, is the development of premade packets of written information including educational materials in multiple languages, which patients can review prior and subsequent to testing.[19]

ENSURING LINKAGE TO CARE

One of the most important components of any ED HIV screening program is ensuring that the patients who test positive are brought into the health care system for ongoing care and monitoring of their HIV. Earlier initiation of medical care for HIV is one of the primary goals of ED screening. Unfortunately, the ED is a difficult venue from which to ensure ongoing care through the medical system. Patients are frequently told to secure outpatient follow-up for a variety of illnesses by their emergency physician, but the numbers who are compliant with these recommendations are often small. When a patient is diagnosed with a positive rapid HIV test in the ED, the need for follow-up is imperative to ensure that confirmatory results are provided and ongoing care is initiated.[20]

While many studies have been done to determine the feasibility of HIV screening in the ED from an operational standpoint, fewer have documented their success in terms of the number of patients who tested positive and were successfully linked to care. In 2007, *Morbidity and Mortality Weekly Report* published results from 3 ED-based HIV screening programs regarding their success, and provided information regarding linkage to care. All 3 programs reviewed had HIV counselors actively involved to maximize the number of patients who attended their follow-up appointments. In all 3 cases, appointment slots were available at local HIV clinics for patients with preliminary positive results in the ED. All confirmatory tests were sent while the patient was still in the ED, and results were available at the time of the follow-up appointment. While the range of successful follow-up varied from 79% to 91%, the overall rate of care linkage was 88% when pooling data from all 3 programs. The most successful ED-based linkage to care was accomplished at Highland Hospital, where dedicated appointment slots were provided at a set time each week by the HIV outpatient clinic for preliminary positives from the ED. A linkage coordinator from that clinic was primarily responsible for facilitating outpatient follow-up for these patients. On average, the time between initial ED diagnosis of HIV and initiation of follow-up care for the patients in this program was 14 days.[7,12]

In most established HIV screening programs, linkage to care is accomplished by combining the efforts of an HIV counselor who encourages and facilitates patient follow-up with the presence of dedicated weekly appointment slots at the closest HIV clinic.[7,12,20,21] Other tactics employed to increase rates of follow-up include contacting patients by phone before their first follow-up appointment, providing an opportunity for the patient to speak with an HIV provider either by phone or in person at the time of the preliminary diagnosis, and ensuring clinic appointments within 24 hours of the preliminary diagnosis. Although the value of these interventions is not clearly proven, they serve as a starting point in the effort to increase rates of linkage to care among newly diagnosed ED patients.[22]

BARRIERS TO ESTABLISHING AN ED-BASED HIV SCREENING PROGRAM

Although the CDC has recommended HIV screening in EDs, many of those who have tried to initiate testing within these guidelines have confronted numerous barriers and obstacles. In CDC-based focus groups and surveys, emergency practitioners noted a lack of time during the patient encounter, inability to ensure follow-up care, lack of privacy in the ED, language and cultural barriers, and the cost of testing as some of the primary reasons that HIV screening was not offered in their EDs.[11] Taking these identified problems into account, the CDC attempted to improve the feasibility of HIV screening in the ED by shortening the time required for obtaining consent and providing pre-/posttest counseling. There are still significant issues of manpower, cost, and staff buy-in that have been at the forefront of recent discussions about HIV screening programs.[7,13,20,22–24] As a result, the reality is that ED HIV screening is rarely performed outside of academic or research settings, which may provide additional support for this type of initiative.[7]

The example of Highland Hospital's ED screening program illustrates many of the manpower difficulties commonly encountered. In this program, an attempt was made to incorporate HIV screening using existing ED staff. All patients who met screening guidelines were supposed to be offered HIV testing at the time of triage by the triage nurse, with streamlined consent being obtained in an opt-in fashion simultaneously. Pretest counseling consisted of a preprinted brochure offered to the patient. HIV counselors were not used in any way in this model. The results of this project demonstrated that only 38.2% of patients were offered testing, and less than 10% actually ended up being screened. Project coordinators found that triage nurses were not offering screening in many cases. Although 10% of patients were deemed ineligible, further analysis revealed that in 44% of cases nurses failed to offer HIV screening. Reasons cited for this included the triage nurse's perception that certain patients were not at risk for HIV, the triage nurse being too busy, concerns regarding patient privacy, and a lack of triage nurse training.[7,13] The benefit of this type of program is its ability to offer 24-hour ED HIV screening without hiring additional staff or relying on staff from another department. Difficulties encountered included the failure of ED staff to incorporate offering HIV screening into the triage process for all eligible patients, the required additional training for ED staff offering and performing the HIV tests, the time required to oversee the program and point-of-care laboratory quality assurance process, and the reliance on funds from an external source for the rapid testing kits.[7] External sources of funds could include the state department of health, private grants, or charitable donations.

In contrast to the Highland Hospital program, George Washington University attempted to develop an ED-based HIV screening program that relied completely on undergraduate students trained in HIV counseling and testing as manpower. HIV screening was available for ED patients from 8 AM to midnight on a daily basis, rather than 24 hours, as the additional staff was only available at those times. During times of increased volumes, 2 screeners were staffed. Data from this program focuses primarily on issues of cost. Each screener was estimated to cost the department $7.50 per hour and each testing kit had an estimated cost of $12. Based on this information and the number of patients screened, the calculated cost per preliminary positive test was estimated at $1700. When including the cost of confirmatory testing, the cost per HIV-positive case rose to $4900. The authors of this study emphasize that this type of intervention is cost-effective based on these numbers, but recognize that billing insurers for HIV screening is a key component to the cost feasibility of screening programs that has yet to be established.[22] Although billing codes have been developed for rapid HIV testing, it remains unclear whether third-party payers will reimburse EDs for those charges.[20] Other studies evaluating the cost-effectiveness of HIV screening have shown a cost of $35,000 to $65,000 per quality-adjusted year (QALY) gained, as compared with screening for other diseases, such as diabetes ($70,000 per QALY gained) and hypertension ($80,000 per QALY gained), which have shown greater costs and are done on a routine basis.[22]

Expense and savings are key issues that arise in the debate regarding the value of HIV screening in the ED. Performing a cost analysis of a proposed HIV screening program is essential to convincing administrators as well as funding sources of the program's value. In one analysis, the costs of conventional HIV testing were compared with rapid HIV testing in the ED and an STD clinic. The investigators noted that although the cost of running an HIV test using a rapid testing kit was higher, the cost of ensuring correct notification of results was lower among those using the rapid kit in an ED setting. Weighing those factors in the analysis, the investigators concluded that the per-patient cost of rapid testing and notification in the ED was lower than in an STD clinic or using conventional testing as long as the proportion of patients accepting the test was greater than 15%. In their analysis of the cost per HIV-infected patient receiving a result, the ED screening program using rapid testing was shown to be the lowest cost, given that the cost of the rapid testing kit remained less than $11. An important point regarding the cost of any screening program is that the exact cost/benefit ratio varies based on the prevalence of the disease in the tested population. The numbers from this study were used to demonstrate that HIV screening in a population with a 0.2% prevalence of HIV has been shown to cost up to $8000 per HIV-infected patient, versus a cost of between $300 and $900 per HIV-infected patient given all of the same variables in a population with 5.4% HIV prevalence. Overall, this analysis demonstrated the value of ED-based rapid HIV screening programs in higher prevalence populations as compared with more traditional STD clinic–based HIV testing programs from a financial perspective.[23]

Aside from cost and manpower issues, securing buy-in from the hospital staff, including nurses, physicians, laboratory technicians, and social workers, is essential to the success of any ED-based program. In preparation for the implementation of an HIV screening program, many recommend identifying an HIV screening supporter or "champion," from each group of staff involved in the process. Ideally an emergency physician and emergency nurse "champion" would lead the efforts to educate staff regarding the screening program, to emphasize importance of conducting screening in a standardized fashion, to assist with smoothing out implementation difficulties as they arise, and to solicit feedback. As HIV screening in the ED is a huge coordinated effort by multiple levels of staff, awareness of its purpose helps to obtain buy-in from an already overworked staff. In addition to the ED staff, hospital administrators and infectious disease providers should be directly involved in the implementation and efforts to sustain HIV screening in the ED.[20]

Another important step in establishing HIV screening in the ED is ensuring that results are delivered and recorded. A review of programs already in existence shows that the delivery of HIV-negative results can successfully be accomplished by HIV counselors, nurses, physicians, or social workers. The published experiences of most of these programs demonstrates the importance of preliminary positive results being reported by the physician or HIV counselor assigned to that patient. Support from nursing staff and social work staff is beneficial in these cases as well. The greater challenge has proven to be ensuring that the preliminary positive or negative result becomes part of the medical record so that future health care providers have access to that information. Ideally, this could be accomplished by incorporating the result into the computerized medical record for that patient, but in practice many programs have found this difficult to accomplish.[20]

SUMMARY

Although some of the aforementioned hurdles to developing an HIV screening program within the ED may seem considerable, CDC officials, state health department staff, and ED staff continue to pursue the goal of early identification of unknown HIV-infected patients through HIV screening programs in the ED. The value of early identification and treatment of HIV-infected patients is clear, but the most effective method for accomplishing this has yet to be determined. Throughout this article, published experiences by ED-based HIV screening programs have been reviewed to learn lessons from their mistakes and accomplishments. The goal of this article is to encourage thought regarding previous experiences with HIV screening and future ideas for improving efforts to this end. By examining the variety of HIV testing kits available, the debate regarding targeted testing versus screening, the consent and patient education requirements, and the staffing models used to implement HIV testing in the ED, this review aims to provide ED physicians and administrators with options that can be tailored based on the resources available in their specific venue. Ultimately, any universal recommendation will have to be adjusted to the local environment in which is it implemented. As the information presented in this article demonstrates, the feasibility and cost-effectiveness of developing an ED-based HIV screening program depends on multiple institution-specific factors including the prevalence of HIV in the population served, as well as the availability of additional funds and staff to ensure its success. Although the goal of HIV screening in all acute care settings set out by the CDC has not been realized, strides continue in pursuit of this end, with a significant amount of learning along the way.

REFERENCES

1. CDC. Revised recommendations for HIV testing of adults, adolescents, and pregnant women in health-care settings. MMWR Morb Mortal Wkly Rep 2006; 55(R-14):1–17.
2. Lyss SB, Branson BM, Kroc KA, et al. Detecting unsuspected HIV infection with a rapid whole blood HIV test in an urban emergency department. J Acquir Immune Defic Syndr 2007;44(4):435–42.
3. Ehrenkranz PD, Ahn CJ, Metlay JP, et al. Availability of rapid HIV testing in academic emergency departments. Acad Emerg Med 2008;15:144–50.
4. CDC. FDA-approved rapid HIV antibody screening tests. Available at: http://www.cdc.gov/hiv/topics/testing/rapid/rt-comparison.htm. Accessed August 2, 2009.
5. Branson BM. HIV screening in health care settings: new approaches and new paradigms. Centers for Disease Control and Prevention, Strategic Planning Workshop for Hospitals. Washington, DC, 2008.
6. Zetola NM, Kaplan B, Dowling T, et al. Prevalence and correlates of unknown HIV infection among patients seeking care in a public hospital emergency department. Public Health Rep 2008;123(Suppl 3):41–51.

7. White DAE, Scribner AN, Schulden JD, et al. Results of a rapid HIV screening and diagnostic testing program in an urban emergency department. Ann Emerg Med 2009;54(1):56–64.

8. Brown J, Kuo I, Bellows J, et al. Patient perceptions and acceptance of routine emergency department HIV testing. Public Health Rep 2008;123(Suppl 3):21–6.

9. Merchant RC, Seage GR, Mayer KH, et al. Emergency department patient acceptance of opt-in, universal rapid HIV screening. Public Health Rep 2008;123(Suppl 3):27–40.

10. Rothman RE. Current centers for disease control and prevention guidelines for HIV counseling, testing and referral: critical role of and a call to action for emergency physicians. Ann Emerg Med 2004;44:31–42.

11. Jenkins TC, Gardner EM, Thurn MW, et al. Risk-based HIV testing fails to detect the majority of HIV infected persons in medical care settings. Sex Transm Dis 2006;33(5):329–33.

12. CDC. Rapid HIV testing in emergency departments—three U.S. sites, January 2005-March 2006. MMWR Morb Mortal Wkly Rep 2007;56(24):597–601.

13. White DA, Warren OU, Scribner AN, et al. Missed opportunities for earlier HIV diagnosis in an emergency department despite an HIV screening program. AIDS Patient Care STDS 2009;23(4):245–52.

14. Haukoos JS, Hopkins E, Byyny RL, et al. Patient acceptance of rapid HIV testing practices in an urban emergency department: assessment of the 2006 CDC recommendations for HIV screening in health care settings. Ann Emerg Med 2008;51(3):303–9.

15. Silverman M, Haukoos JS. HIV testing in the emergency department: pretest counseling or pretest education. Ann Emerg Med 2007;49(5):380.

16. Merchant RC, Clark MA, Mayer KH, et al. Video as an effective method to deliver pretest information for rapid HIV testing. Acad Emerg Med 2009;16:124–35.

17. Calderon Y, Haughley M, Bijur PE, et al. An educational HIV pretest counseling video program for off-hours testing in the emergency department. Ann Emerg Med 2006;48(1):21–7.

18. Calderon Y, Leider J, Hailpern S, et al. A randomized control trial evaluating the educational effectiveness of a rapid HIV post-test counseling video. Sex Transm Dis 2009;36(4):207–10.

19. Lyons MS, Christopher LJ, Ledyard HK, et al. Emergency department HIV testing and counseling: an ongoing experience in a low-prevalence area. Ann Emerg Med 2005;46(1):22–8.

20. Brown J, Shesser R, Simon G. Establishing an ED HIV screening program: lessons from the front lines. Acad Emerg Med 2007;14(7):658–61.

21. Gift TL, Hogben M. Emergency department STD and HIV screening: findings from a national survey. Acad Emerg Med 2006;13(9):993.

22. Brown J, Shesser R, Simon G, et al. Routine HIV screening in the emergency department using the new United States centers for disease control and prevention guidelines. J Acquir Immune Defic Syndr 2007;46(4):395–401.

23. Farnham PG, Hutchinson AB, Sanson SL, et al. Comparing the costs of HIV screening strategies and technologies in health care settings. Public Health Rep 2008;123(Suppl 3):51–62.

24. Silva A, Glick NR, Lyss SB, et al. Implementing an HIV and STD screening program in an ED. Ann Emerg Med 2007;49(5):564–72.

Acute HIV Infection: Diagnosis and Management in the Emergency Department

Wesley H. Self, MD[a,b],*

KEYWORDS

- HIV • AIDS • Acute retroviral syndrome
- Emergency department

EPIDEMIOLOGY

Mathematical modeling and epidemiologic studies suggest that infection in a large proportion of new cases of human immunodeficiency virus (HIV) are contracted from people with acute HIV infection.[1–3] There are several factors that cause the period of acute HIV infection to be one of high infectivity; these include high viral loads in the blood and genital secretions, patients' unawareness of being infected with HIV, and patients continuing the risky behavior, including unprotected sex and needle sharing, that led to their own recent infection.

Most patients with acute HIV infection experience a symptomatic episode with a sudden-onset viral illness. Many of these patients seek medical attention in emergency departments (EDs) and primary care clinics.[4,5] Therefore, recognizing acute HIV infection in the ED and initiating strategies to prevent further transmission are important opportunities to limit the spread of HIV.

PATHOPHYSIOLOGY

On a cellular level, infection involves the HIV envelope glycoprotein (gp) 120 binding to the CD4 receptor on human T cells, macrophages, and dendritic cells. After

Support: This material is based on work supported by the Office of Academic Affiliations, Department of Veterans Affairs, Veterans Affairs National Quality Scholars Program, and with resources and the use of facilities at Veterans Affairs Tennessee Valley Healthcare System, Nashville, Tennessee.

Disclosures: The author has no disclosures to report.

[a] Department of Emergency Medicine, Vanderbilt University, 1313, 21st Avenue South, 703 Oxford House, Nashville, TN 37232, USA

[b] Tennessee Valley Healthcare System, Veterans Health Administration, 1310 24th Avenue South, Nashville, TN 37212, USA

* Department of Emergency Medicine, Vanderbilt University, 1313, 21st Avenue South, 703 Oxford House, Nashville, TN 37232.

E-mail address: wesley.self@vanderbilt.edu

Emerg Med Clin N Am 28 (2010) 381–392
doi:10.1016/j.emc.2010.01.002
0733-8627/10/$ – see front matter. Published by Elsevier Inc.

a conformational change in gp120, it binds a coreceptor, either CCR5 or CXCR4, on the cellular membrane, allowing entry into these human cells.[6] The virus then replicates, leading to cellular death in the infected cells and nearby bystander immune cells.[7] Acute infection is marked by massive viral replication in an environment rich in $CD4^+$, $CCR5^+$, and $CXCR4^+$ target cells and unchecked by the host immune system, which has not been previously sensitized to HIV antigens.

HIV infection most commonly occurs by sexual transmission through the genital mucosa. At the time of sexual contact, viral particles cross the mucous membrane and enter the $CD4^+$ dendritic cells. The virus then spreads locally to other $CD4^+$ cells, and by 72 hours it establishes infection at the site of inoculation and the draining lymph tissue.[8] After 7 days, the virus has disseminated systemically via the lymph system and blood and is detectable in peripheral blood by nucleic acid amplification testing (NAAT), such as a viral load measurement.[9,10] Days 8 to 30 after infection are characterized by massive viral replication, with a doubling of the viral load approximately every 8 hours, and the death of large numbers of $CD4^+$ cells.[11,12] Intestinal $CD4^+$ cells in the gut-associated lymphoid tissue are severely depleted, leading to a whole-body loss of $CD4^+$ cells that is more profound than is reflected in the peripheral blood CD4 count.[10,13] During this time, the host's immune system is broadly activated, leading to the symptoms of acute retroviral syndrome. The intense immune activation may be provoked by translocation of gut bacteria through the intestinal immune barrier that has been damaged by HIV.[14] The immune system begins to mount an HIV-specific response, and the first anti-HIV antibodies are produced. Using standard third-generation enzyme immunoassays (EIAs) available in clinical practice, HIV antibodies can typically first be detected in a patient's serum 3 to 7 weeks postinfection, marking the event of seroconversion (**Fig. 1**).[15]

Peak levels of viremia and genital shedding occur around day 30, followed by a period of precipitous decline in viral load 4 to 10 weeks postinfection. The causes for this decline in viremia are incompletely understood but likely involve the depletion of the reservoir of $CD4^+$ or $CCR5^+$ cells available for infection and the appearance of specific anti-HIV $CD8^+$ cytotoxic lymphocytes that limit viral replication.[16,17] Week 10 represents the nadir of viral load and genital secretions. Weeks 10 to 24 are characterized by an interplay between the host immune response and viral replication, eventually leading to a point of equilibrium with a stable viral load and CD4 count, termed the set point.[18] Although the terminology has not been standardized, week 24 is typically considered the end of acute HIV infection, after which the patient enters the period of chronic HIV infection.

CLINICAL FEATURES

The clinical manifestations of acute HIV infection, commonly called acute retroviral syndrome, were first described in 1985 as an acute mononucleosis-like illness occurring before seroconversion.[19] The syndrome has since been well characterized. There is typically an incubation period of 10 to 14 days before the onset of symptoms, which variably include fever, malaise, myalgias, arthralgias, night sweats, headache, sore throat, nausea, vomiting, anorexia, and weight loss.[4,5,20,21] Fever and malaise are the most common symptoms, with each being present in more than 70% of cases.[22] When gastrointestinal symptoms are present, anorexia and weight loss are usually prominent. The headache is often described as retrobulbar pain exacerbated with eye movements.

Possible physical examination findings include a generalized lymphadenopathy, often most pronounced in the axillary, cervical, and occipital nodes[23]; modest

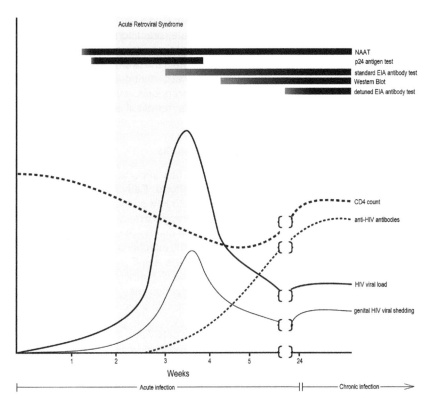

Fig. 1. Dynamics of HIV viral load, host CD4 count, and host expression of anti-HIV antibodies during acute HIV infection. The shaded region represents the usual timing and duration of acute retroviral syndrome. The bars demonstrate when during HIV infection the named diagnostic tests are typically positive. (*Adapted from* Zetola NM, Pilcher CD. Diagnosis and management of acute HIV infection. Infect Dis Clin N Am 2007;21:22; with permission and *Data from* Fiebig EW, Wright DJ, Rawal BD, et al. Dynamics of HIV viremia and antibody seroconversion in plasma donors: implications for diagnosis and staging of primary HIV infection. AIDS 2003;17:1876; with permission.)

hepatosplenomegaly; oral/vaginal thrush; pharyngeal erythema and edema without exudates[24]; rash; and mucocutaneous ulcers. A small red maculopapular rash appears on the upper thorax, face, scalp, and limbs, including the palms and soles; it typically starts 2 to 3 days after the onset of fever and persists for 5 to 8 days.[25] The mucocutaneous ulcers are shallow, sharply demarked lesions that occur in the mouth, esophagus, anus, and genitalia, with a propensity for sites of sexual contact.[25] Abnormalities on routine laboratory test results are nonspecific and potentially seen in other acute viral illnesses; these include mild anemia, leukopenia, thrombocytopenia, and transaminitis.[26] Opportunistic infections, including pneumocystis pneumonia, and severe neurologic disease, such as HIV encephalitis, have been reported but are rare during acute infection.[27] Most signs and symptoms of acute HIV infection last for approximately 7 to 10 days, with the exception of malaise, lymphadenopathy, mucocutaneous ulcers, and laboratory abnormalities, which can persist for months.[20]

It is difficult to precisely determine the percentage of people with acute HIV who are symptomatic. This difficulty stems from asymptomatic patients rarely seeking medical attention and symptomatic patients rarely being diagnosed with HIV due to the nonspecific, self-resolving nature of the symptoms, practitioners failing to consider acute HIV as a potential cause of a severe viral illness, and rapid HIV tests giving negative results during the period of acute infection. Within these limitations, it is estimated that as many as 90% of patients are symptomatic during acute infection.[4,5] The severity of symptoms correlates with long-term prognosis, with patients manifesting more extensive and severe symptoms of acute retroviral syndrome progressing more quickly to AIDS.[28]

RATIONALE FOR PURSUING AN ACUTE HIV DIAGNOSIS

Establishing a diagnosis of acute HIV infection has important implications for the individual patient, public health, and research efforts. Early diagnosis enables the HIV-infected patient to establish a relationship with HIV specialists, enter a disease-monitoring program, and begin antiretroviral therapy (ART) and prophylaxis against opportunistic infections at optimal times. When the diagnosis is not made in the acute phase it is often delayed for years until opportunistic infections develop.[29,30] Because of this delay, patients lose the opportunity for the significant survival benefits of starting ART in the pre-AIDS phase of the disease.[31] Furthermore, there is growing evidence that initiating ART during acute HIV infection may improve reconstitution of the immune system, although the long-term clinical effects of early antiretroviral treatment are still unknown.[32]

From a public health standpoint, early diagnosis of HIV maximizes the opportunities to prevent the spread of infection through patient education on practicing abstinence or safe sex, avoiding needle sharing, and avoiding blood donation. If the diagnosis is delayed, HIV-infected people may infect many others during their acute infection, which is the period of greatest infectious potential due to high levels of viral shedding and viremia.[33] Wawer and colleagues[34] found that the rate of HIV transmission per sexual contact was 10 times higher during the first 5 months of infection compared with chronic infections in HIV-discordant couples. Without intervention, patients who recently contracted HIV are likely to transmit the virus to others by engaging in the same risky behavior that led to their own infection.[35] Indeed, epidemiologic studies and mathematical modeling suggest that a substantial proportion of all HIV infections are likely contracted from people with an acute HIV infection.[1–3] Therefore, a diagnosis of acute HIV represents an important opportunity to intervene on the transmission of the virus and potentially prevent an outbreak of HIV.

From a research perspective, identification of acute HIV cases enables scientists to investigate the best preventative strategies and treatment options for early infection and to accurately monitor trends in HIV transmission.

IDENTIFYING WHO TO TEST

Acute HIV infection is a challenging diagnosis to make. It is rarely diagnosed even when a patient presents with an identifiable risk factor for HIV and symptoms of acute retroviral syndrome.[5] One challenge is identifying which patients among those presenting with an acute viral illness should undergo HIV testing. The prevalence of acute HIV among patients presenting to the ED with an acute febrile illness is likely higher than what most emergency physicians recognize. Rosenberg and colleagues[36] retrospectively tested blood samples for HIV from 563 patients who were tested for mononucleosis with a heterophil antibody test at an institution in Boston during a 1-year period. They found that 1.2% of these patients had test results consistent with acute HIV infection. Similarly, Pincus and colleagues[37] tested 499 patients who presented to a Boston urgent care center during a 1-year period with any symptoms of a viral illness and a risk factor for HIV and found a 1.0% prevalence of acute HIV infection. No combination of signs and symptoms reliably distinguishes patients with acute HIV infection from other viral illnesses[20,37]; therefore, liberal use of HIV testing among patients with signs of potential acute HIV infection and risk factors for the disease is warranted.

In 2006, the Centers for Disease Control and Prevention (CDC) revised its recommendations on HIV testing and now advocates routine HIV screening in all health care settings, including the ED.[38] To alleviate previous barriers to routine HIV testing, the CDC also recommends that separate written consent and prevention counseling should not be required before HIV testing.

All patients presenting with an acute, febrile illness in the ED should be questioned about HIV risk factors, including a suspected or known HIV-infected sexual partner, a history of sexually transmitted diseases, multiple sexual partners, receptive anal intercourse, active genital ulcer in self or partner, traumatic sex, intravenous drug use, needle sharing, or recent occupational blood exposure.[39–41] Specific questioning and physical examination should target the clinical features that are more common in HIV than in other viral illnesses; these include weight loss, lack of nasal congestion, generalized lymphadenopathy, oral/genital/anal ulcerations, a diffuse rash involving the palms and soles, and an illness severe enough to lead to hospitalization.[20–22] Patients with an acute febrile viral syndrome plus a risk factor for HIV should undergo testing for acute HIV infection. Patients with clinical features that are more common in acute HIV than in other viral illnesses but no clearly identified risk factor for HIV should be considered for acute HIV testing.

Testing for mononucleosis and influenza can be helpful in establishing an alternative diagnosis before pursuing testing for acute HIV. However, the heterophil antibody test result is occasionally positive during acute HIV infection. Whether this represents a false-positive test or a concurrent infection with HIV and Epstein-Barr virus is not known.[42]

DIAGNOSTIC TESTING

When pursuing a diagnosis of acute HIV infection, emergency physicians should either test for HIV or arrange for prompt inpatient or outpatient testing. Testing practices vary among institutions depending on the availability of HIV diagnostic tests; each ED should develop a protocol to facilitate timely testing, whether it is completed in the department or after referral.

Two classes of HIV tests are important when considering acute infection: serologic tests, which detect antibodies produced by the patient in response to HIV infection, and NAATs, which detect viral RNA within the patient's blood. Standard serologic testing for HIV involves an EIA test, followed by a confirmatory Western blot assay if the result of EIA is positive. For the results of serologic tests to be considered positive, the CDC requires that antibodies to at least 2 of the following antigens be detected: p24, p41, and gp120. Results are reported as positive, negative, or indeterminate. Indeterminate results usually result from a positive EIA and detection of a single antibody, usually anti-p24, on Western blot; this can occur during the period of partial seroconversion during acute HIV infection.

A positive serologic test result is the standard for diagnosing chronic HIV infection. However, serologic testing alone is unreliable for acute infection because of the time lag between inoculation and seroconversion, historically called the diagnostic window. By using the third-generation EIA in today's clinical practice, it has been found that seroconversion typically occurs 3 to 7 weeks after infection.[15] It is a common misconception that serologic testing cannot detect HIV infection before

24 weeks. Twenty-four weeks after a potential HIV exposure, the sensitivity for serologic testing is greater than 95%; thus, completing serologic testing after 24 weeks of exposure is often recommended when trying to exclude infection.[43] However, antibodies can be detected as early as 3 weeks in many patients, and a positive serologic test result does not exclude acute HIV infection in symptomatic patients.

Similar to EIA, rapid HIV tests, which screen for HIV antibodies by applying patient specimens to a membrane affixed with HIV antigens, require Western blot confirmation after a positive test result and do not rule out acute infection with a negative result.[44]

A less-sensitive, detuned EIA test has been developed to distinguish chronic infection from acute infection among patients with positive results from standard serologic testing.[45] The detuned EIA HIV test is available from the CDC and some research laboratories. The sensitivity of this test is reduced by diluting the samples and decreasing incubation times so that the result becomes positive approximately 24 weeks after infection.[46] Therefore, a negative result from detuned EIA with a concurrent positive result from more sensitive tests, such as NAAT, standard serology, or rapid serology, suggests acute infection with inoculation within the previous 24 weeks.

NAAT refers to any test that detects viral genetic material from patient specimens. Both qualitative and quantitative NAATs have been developed for the detection of HIV RNA. The quantitative test, commonly called the viral load, is typically performed using reverse transcriptase–polymerase chain reaction technology. It can detect as few as 40 copies/mL and shows positive results in the first or second week of infection.[47] When patients develop acute retroviral syndrome, they have very high viral loads, usually greater than 100,000 copies/mL.[21] Therefore, NAATs are the standard for diagnosing HIV infection during the acute phase. False-positive results in NAATs occur in 3% to 5% of patients, depending on the disease prevalence but are usually recognizable by a low viral load (<10,000 copies/mL) that is inconsistent with acute infection.[20]

The diagnosis of acute HIV infection is made by a positive NAAT plus serologic test result consistent with acute infection, with results that are either negative for standard serology testing or indeterminate or positive for standard serologic testing with a negative results for detuned serologic test (**Table 1**). At present, NAATs require several hours to complete; furthermore, for screening tests, qualitative NAATs are often pooled to reduce costs.[48] Therefore, a diagnosis of acute HIV infection cannot be confirmed by NAAT in the time frame of a typical ED patient course. When acute

Table 1
The results of diagnostic tests during acute and chronic HIV infection

	No HIV Infection	Acute HIV Infection	Chronic HIV Infection
Serologic Testing (standard and rapid)	Neg	Usually neg[a]	Pos
Detuned Serology	Neg	Neg	Pos
NAAT	Neg	Pos	Pos
p24 Antigen Test	Neg	Pos	Pos or neg

Abbreviations: Neg, negative; Pos, positive.
[a] Standard serologic and rapid serologic test results are usually negative during acute HIV infection; however, because of the high sensitivity of modern serologic tests and the ability to detect some immature IgM antibodies, serologic tests are rarely positive or indeterminate.

HIV infection is considered, the emergency physician should either order an NAAT and arrange for the patient to obtain the results or arrange for close follow-up, whereby an NAAT can be performed.

Assays that detect the HIV p24 antigen are an alternative to NAATs for diagnosing acute HIV infection. The p24 antigen test result becomes positive 3 to 6 days after performing NAATs and is technically simpler. However, the p24 test is less sensitive than NAATs and cannot be pooled, and the result is not reliably positive during chronic infection; less than half of the patients with chronic HIV infection have a positive p24 antigen test result because of patient antibodies binding the p24 antigen and interfering with the test.[21,49] Therefore, nucleic acid testing is typically preferred over the p24 antigen test for diagnosing acute infection.

MANAGEMENT

A 4-pronged approach to the treatment of acute HIV infection involves considering the initiation of ART, arranging long-term care with an HIV specialist, decreasing the risk of further transmission through patient counseling, and providing psychosocial support. Given the uncertainties of ART for acute HIV infection and the clear benefits of close, long-term care, consultation with an HIV specialist immediately on diagnosing acute HIV infection is recommended. Ideally, the emergency physician and HIV specialist would discuss whether to initiate immediate ART and how to establish follow-up care for the patient.

ART

The decision whether to treat any HIV-positive patient with ART requires a careful consideration of potential benefits and costs of treatment for that patient. The long-term clinical effects of antiretroviral treatment during the acute phase of HIV infection have not been well elucidated, making management decisions particularly challenging during acute infection.[31,32] It is hoped that ongoing studies will improve the understanding of the effects of ART during acute infection[50]; however, it remains a challenging subject to study due to the rarity with which HIV is diagnosed before seroconversion.

Preliminary studies indicate that there may be some benefit to starting ART as soon as possible during acute infection. These benefits potentially include protecting CD4$^+$ cells early in the infection, allowing a more robust initial anti-HIV immune response[51]; limiting viral mutations and therefore decreasing the potential for antiviral resistance; improving the symptoms of acute retroviral syndrome; and decreasing the risk of viral transmission during peak levels of viremia.[22,52] Potential costs of early ART include increased medication toxicity due to exposure to the agents for longer periods and the substantial financial costs of the medications. Furthermore, early ART may drive antiviral resistance if the medications do not completely suppress viral replication, which is particularly a problem if patients are poorly compliant with the medication regimen.

Studies examining early ART around the time of seroconversion followed by cessation of treatment have had mixed results, with some studies suggesting benefits in disease progression, CD4 counts, and viral loads[53-56] and others showing no benefit from early-initiated, interrupted antiretroviral treatment.[57-59] Patients with the highest likelihood to benefit from immediate ART may be those with severe, unremitting symptoms of acute retroviral syndrome and those with an initial CD4 count less than 350 cells/μL.[22] A theoretical benefit of starting continuous ART during acute HIV infection is maximal control of the infection while new, more effective therapies are developed. Aggressive treatment may delay progression of the infection and thus preserve treatment options if a more effective, and perhaps even curative, treatment emerges in the future.[32]

Long-term Treatment

Establishing a protocol for the acutely infected patient to receive long-term HIV care is an essential component of initial management. Establishing care in an HIV clinic is important for proper disease monitoring, preventative measures such as immunizations and prophylactic antibiotics, initiating and altering ART regimens, and ongoing counseling. Ideally, a patient with acute HIV infection would also be enrolled in one of the ongoing HIV clinical trials to help enhance the understanding of acute infection and optimal treatment strategies.

Public Health Interventions

Acute HIV infection is a public health emergency and is an opportunity for the emergency physician to help prevent further transmission. With assistance of the local public health department, a potential source of the patient's HIV infection and all recent high-risk contacts may be identified. By following the syphilis elimination model that the public health strategy used to limit syphilis transmission, the index patient's network of sexual and needle contacts can be identified, screened for HIV, and given risk reduction counseling.[60] The goal is to identify a network of people at risk for HIV infection and interrupt ongoing transmission of the disease. Risk reduction counseling should be initiated immediately in every patient diagnosed with HIV; such counseling should consist of clear education about the infectious potential of acute HIV and strategies to prevent its spread, including practicing sexual abstinence, using condoms, avoiding needle sharing, and not donating blood. Brief risk reduction counseling has been shown to greatly reduce risky behavior that can lead to HIV transmission.[61,62] This counseling seems to be particularly effective for patients who recently tested positive for HIV.[63]

During an HIV screening program in North Carolina between November 2002 and October 2004, 44 people were identified as having acute HIV infection.[48,60] These 44 people reported a total of 130 named and 69 anonymous sexual partners in the previous 6 months. About 78%of the named partners were successfully notified as being high risk for HIV; 67% of the partners not previously known to be HIV positive agreed to HIV testing, and 39% tested HIV positive. The likely source patient was identified and counseled in 56% of cases. The success of this program demonstrates that after a diagnosis of acute HIV infection is established, a network of people with contact to the index case who are at high risk for HIV can be rapidly identified, tested, and counseled.

Psychosocial Support

Being diagnosed with acute HIV infection is extremely distressing and is often accompanied by other psychosocial stressors, including drug use and psychiatric illness.[64,65] Patients with recent HIV diagnoses are often concerned about their privacy and are further distressed by repeated questioning about their sexual practices and drug habits. Therefore, psychosocial counseling is an essential component of the management of acute HIV. Involvement of social workers, psychologists, and psychiatrists as needed during the initial evaluation is encouraged.

SUMMARY

Acute HIV infection is difficult to recognize in the ED but is a relatively common and highly damaging disease. The keys to diagnosis are questioning patients with acute febrile illnesses about HIV risk factors and maintaining a low threshold for testing for acute HIV infection. Serologic testing is not sufficient to assess for acute infection;

a test to detect HIV RNA by nucleic acid amplification, which can detect HIV within the first 2 weeks of infection, is recommended. The effects of ART during acute infection have not been clearly established; therefore, consultation with an HIV specialist is recommended when considering antiretroviral treatment. When caring for patients with acute HIV infection, establishing a protocol for them to receive long-term care and psychosocial support and initiating a public health investigation to limit the spread of HIV from these index cases are essential.

ACKNOWLEDGMENTS

I would like to thank Todd Hulgan, MD, MPH, for his helpful comments on the content of this article and Josh Keckley for his assistance with producing the figures.

REFERENCES

1. Pinkerton SD. Probability of HIV transmission during acute infection in Rakai, Uganda. AIDS Behav 2008;12(5):677–84.
2. Jacquez JA, Koopman JS, Simon CP, et al. Role of the primary infection in epidemics of HIV infection in gay cohorts. J Acquir Immune Defic Syndr 1994; 7(11):1169–84.
3. Pilcher CD, Tien HC, Eron JJ, et al. Brief but efficient: acute HIV infection and the sexual transmission of HIV. J Infect Dis 2004;189(10):1785–92.
4. Tindall B, Barker S, Donovan B, et al. Characterization of the acute clinical illness associated with human immunodeficiency virus infection. Arch Intern Med 1988; 148(4):945.
5. Schacker T, Collier AC, Hughes J, et al. Clinical and epidemiologic features of primary HIV infection. Ann Intern Med 1996;125(4):257–64.
6. Rucker J, Doms RW. Chemokine receptors as HIV coreceptors: implications and interactions. AIDS Res Hum Retroviruses 1998;14:S241.
7. Vlahakis SR. Cell death in HIV infection: gp120. In: Badley AD, editor. Cell death during HIV infection. Kindle edition. Boca Raton (FL): Taylor & Francis Group; 2005. p. 95–108.
8. Zhang Z, Schuler T, Zupancic M, et al. Sexual transmission and propagation of SIV and HIV in resting and activated CD4+ T cells. Science 1999;286(5443): 1353–7.
9. Miller CJ, Li Q, Abel K, et al. Propagation and dissemination of infection after vaginal transmission of simian immunodeficiency virus. J Virol 2005;79(14): 9217–27.
10. Li Q, Duan L, Estes JD, et al. Peak SIV replication in resting memory CD4+ T cells depletes gut lamina propria CD4+ T cells. Nature 2005;434:1148–52.
11. Little SJ, McLean AR, Spina CA, et al. Viral dynamics of acute HIV-1 infection. J Exp Med 1999;190(6):841–50.
12. Lindback S, Karlsson AC, Mittler J, et al. Viral dynamics in primary HIV-1 infection. AIDS 2000;14(15):2283–91.
13. Mattapallil JJ, Douek DC, Hill B, et al. Massive infection and loss of memory CD4+ T cells in multiple tissues during acute SIV infection. Nature 2005; 434(7037):1093–7.
14. Brenchley JM, Price DA, Schacker TW, et al. Microbial translocation is a cause of systemic immune activation in chronic HIV infection. Nat Med 2006;12(12): 1365–71.
15. Weber B, Gurtler L, Thorstensson R, et al. Multicenter evaluation of a new fourth generation human immunodeficiency virus screening assay with a sensitive

antigen detection module and high specificity. J Clin Microbiol 2002;40(6): 1938–46.

16. Schmitz JE, Kuroda MJ, Santra S, et al. Control of viremia in simian immunodeficiency virus infection by CD8+ lymphocytes. Science 1999;283:857–60.

17. Koup RA, Safrit JT, Cao Y, et al. Temporal association of cellular immune responses with the initial control of viremia in primary human immunodeficiency virus type 1 syndrome. J Virol 1994;68(7):4650–5.

18. Stafford MA, Corey L, Cao Y, et al. Modeling plasma virus concentration during primary HIV infection. J Theor Biol 2000;203(3):285–301.

19. Cooper DA, Gold J, Maclean P, et al. Acute AIDS retrovirus infection. Definition of a clinical illness associated with seroconversion. Lancet 1985;1(8428):537–40.

20. Hecht FM, Busch MP, Rawal B, et al. Use of laboratory tests and clinical symptoms for identification of primary HIV infection. AIDS 2002;16(8):1119–29.

21. Daar ES, Little S, Pitt J. Diagnosis of primary HIV-1 Infection. Ann Intern Med 2001;134:25–9.

22. Zetola NM, Pilcher CD. Diagnosis and management of acute HIV infection. Infect Dis Clin North Am 2007;21:19–48.

23. Gaines H, von Sydow M, Pehrson PO, et al. Clinical picture of primary HIV infection presenting as a glandular-fever-like illness. BMJ 1988;297(6660): 1363–8.

24. Valle SL. Febrile pharyngitis as the primary sign of HIV infection in a cluster of cases linked by sexual contact. Scand J Infect Dis 1987;19(1):13–7.

25. Lapins J, Gaines H, Lindback S, et al. Skin and mucosal characteristics of symptomatic primary HIV-1 infection. AIDS Patient Care STDS 1997;11(2):67–70.

26. Kassutto S, Rosenberg ES. Primary HIV type 1 infection. Clin Infect Dis 2004; 38(10):1447–53.

27. Carne CA, Tedder RS, Smith A, et al. Acute encephalopathy coincident with seroconversion for anti-HTLV-III. Lancet 1985;2(8466):1206–8.

28. Dorrucci M, Rezza G, Vlahov D, et al. Clinical characteristics and prognostic value of acute retroviral syndrome among injecting drug users. AIDS 1995;9(6): 597–604.

29. Keruly JC, Moore RD. Immune status at presentation to care did not improve among antiretroviral-naive persons from 1990 to 2006. Clin Infect Dis 2007; 45(10):1369–74.

30. Brodie S, Sax P. Novel approaches to HIV antibody testing. AIDS Clin Care 1997; 9(1):1–5.

31. Hammer SM, Saag MS, Schechter M, et al. Treatment for adult HIV infection: 2006 recommendations of the international AIDS society—USA panel. JAMA 2006;296: 827–43.

32. Smith DE, Walker BD, Cooper DA, et al. Is antiretroviral treatment of primary HIV infection clinically justified on the basis of current evidence? AIDS 2004;18: 709–18.

33. Pilcher CD, Shugars DC, Fiscus SA, et al. HIV in body fluids during primary HIV infection: implications for pathogenesis, treatment and public health. AIDS 2001; 15(7):837–45.

34. Wawer MJ, Gray RH, Sewankambo NK, et al. Rates of HIV-1 transmission per coital act, by stage of HIV-1 infection, in Rakai, Uganda. J Infect Dis 2005; 191(9):1403–9.

35. Colfax GN, Buchbinder SP, Cornelisse PG, et al. Sexual risk behaviors and implications for secondary HIV transmission during and after HIV seroconversion. AIDS 2002;16:1529–35.

36. Rosenberg ES, Caliendo AM, Walker BD. Acute HIV infection among patients tested for mononucleosis. N Engl J Med 1999;340(12):969.

37. Pincus JM, Crosby SS, Losina E, et al. Acute human immunodeficiency virus infection in patients presenting to an urban urgent care center. Clin Infect Dis 2003;37(12):1699–704.

38. Branson BM, Handsfield HH, Lampe MA, et al. Revised recommendations for HIV testing of adults, adolescents and pregnant women in health-care settings. MMWR Recomm Rep 2006;55(RR14):1–17.

39. Chan DJ. Fatal attraction: sex, sexually transmitted infections and HIV-1. Int J STD AIDS 2006;17(10):643–51.

40. Reynolds SJ, Quinn TC. Developments in STD/HIV interactions: the intertwining epidemics of HIV and HSV-2. Infect Dis Clin North Am 2005;19(2):415–25.

41. Moss AR, Vranizan K, Gorter R, et al. HIV seroconversion in intravenous drug users in San Francisco, 1985–1990. AIDS 1994;8(2):223–31.

42. Vidrih JA, Walensky RP, Sax PE, et al. Positive Epstein-Barr virus heterophile antibody tests in patients with primary human immunodeficiency virus infection. Am J Med 2001;111(3):192–4.

43. Horsburgh CR Jr, Ou CY, Jason J, et al. Duration of human immunodeficiency virus infection before detection of antibody. Lancet 1989;2(8664):637–40.

44. Delaney KP, Branson BM, Uniyal A, et al. Performance of an oral fluid rapid HIV-1/2 test: experience from four CDC studies. AIDS 2006;20(12):1655–60.

45. Janssen RS, Satten GA, Stramer SL, et al. New testing strategy to detect early HIV-1 infection for use in incidence estimates and for clinical and prevention purposes. JAMA 1998;280(1):42–8.

46. Kothe D, Byers RH, Caudill SP, et al. Performance characteristics of a new less sensitive HIV-1 enzyme immunoassay for use in estimating HIV seroincidence. J Acquir Immune Defic Syndr 2003;33(5):625–34.

47. Mulder J, McKinney N, Christopherson C, et al. Rapid and simple PCR assay for quantitation of human immunodeficiency virus type 1 RNA in plasma: application to acute retroviral infection. J Clin Microbiol 1994;32(2):292–300.

48. Pilcher CD, Fiscus SA, Nguyen TQ, et al. Detection of acute infections during HIV testing in North Carolina. N Engl J Med 2005;352(18):1873–83.

49. Schupbach J. Measurement of HIV-1 p24 antigen by signal-amplification-boosted ELISA of heat-denatured plasma is a simple and inexpensive alternative to tests for viral RNA. AIDS Rev 2002;4(2):83–92.

50. Kinloch-de Loes S. Treatment of acute HIV-1 infection: is it coming of age? J Infect Dis 2006;194(6):721–4.

51. Rosenberg ES, Altfeld M, Poon SH, et al. Immune control of HIV-1 after early treatment of acute infection. Nature 2000;407(6803):523–6.

52. Hoen B, Cooper DA, Lampe FC, et al. Predictors of virological outcome and safety in primary HIV type 1-infected patients initiating quadruple antiretroviral therapy: QUEST GW PROB3005. Clin Infect Dis 2007;45(3):381–90.

53. Kinloch-De Loes S, Hirschel BJ, Hoen B, et al. A controlled trial of zidovudine in primary human immunodeficiency virus infection. N Engl J Med 1995;333(7):408–13.

54. Niu MT, Bethel J, Holodniy M, et al. Zidovudine treatment in patients with primary (acute) human immunodeficiency virus type 1 infection: a randomized, double-blind, placebo-controlled trial. J Infect Dis 1998;178(1):80–91.

55. Kassutto S, Maghsoudi K, Johnston MN, et al. Longitudinal analysis of clinical markers following antiretroviral therapy initiated during acute or early HIV type 1 infection. Clin Infect Dis 2006;42(7):1024–31.

56. Hecht FM, Wang L, Collier A, et al. A multicenter observational study of the potential benefits of initiating combination antiretroviral therapy during acute HIV infection. J Infect Dis 2006;194(6):725–33.

57. Streeck H, Jessen H, Alter G, et al. Immunological and virological impact of highly active antiretroviral therapy initiated during acute HIV-1 infection. J Infect Dis 2006;194(6):734–9.

58. Hoen B, Fournier I, Lacabaratz C, et al. Structured treatment interruptions in primary HIV-1 infection: the ANRS 100 PRIMSTOP trial. J Acquir Immune Defic Syndr 2005;40(3):307–16.

59. Pantazis N, Touloumi G, Vanhems P, et al. The effect of antiretroviral treatment of different durations in primary HIV infection. AIDS 2008;22(18):2441–50.

60. Pilcher CD, Eaton L, Kalichman S, et al. Approaching HIV elimination: interventions for acute HIV infection. Curr HIV/AIDS Rep 2006;3(4):160–8.

61. Kamb ML, Fishbein M, Douglas JM, et al. Efficacy of risk-reduction counseling to prevent human immunodeficiency virus and sexually transmitted diseases: a randomized controlled trial. JAMA 1998;280(13):1161–7.

62. Kelly JA, Kalichman SC. Behavioral research in HIV/AIDS primary and secondary prevention: recent advances and future directions. J Consult Clin Psychol 2002; 70(3):626–39.

63. Weinhardt LS, Carey MP, Johnson BT, et al. Effects of HIV counseling and testing on sexual risk behavior: a meta-analytic review of published research, 1985–1997. Am J Public Health 1999;89(9):1397–405.

64. Rabkin JG, Ferrando SJ, Jacobsberg LB, et al. Prevalence of axis I disorders in an AIDS cohort: a cross-sectional, controlled study. Compr Psychiatry 1997; 38(3):146–54.

65. Schrooten W, Dreezen C, Fleerackers Y, et al. Receiving a positive HIV test result: the experience of patients in Europe. HIV Med 2001;2(4):250–4.

Immune Reconstitution Inflammatory Syndrome

George W. Beatty, MD, MPH

KEYWORDS

- Immune reconstitution inflammatory syndrome
- Antiretroviral therapy • Complications of therapy
- Immune restitution disease

With the introduction of potent antiretroviral therapy (ART), patients with HIV infection now achieve restoration of previously compromised immune function, resulting in decreased mortality and morbidity from opportunistic infections. However, as HIV RNA decreases to a very low level, and CD4 count increases, a minority of patients experience apparent paradoxic clinical deterioration as a direct result of this immune restitution. Thus, along with the myriad presentations of opportunistic infections afflicting patients infected with HIV are a group of inflammatory disorders with atypical presentations in patients recently started on ART. This group of disorders, known as immune reconstitution inflammatory syndrome (IRIS) or immune reconstitution disease (IRD), is characterized by an exuberant inflammatory reaction to previously unrecognized or partially treated opportunistic infections. In addition, several autoimmune processes occurring in patients treated with ART have been described, and include de novo presentations of autoimmune disease and flares of preexisting autoimmune disorders.

IRIS poses a diagnostic dilemma to the emergency physician because it occurs in patients who have recently started ART and may have CD4 counts in a range that puts them at risk for a variety of opportunistic infections. IRIS manifests in 2 principal ways. The first of these 2 scenarios occurs when a patient with a previously diagnosed treated infection begins potent ART. As immune restitution ensues, antigens provoke inflammation that causes clinical deterioration despite ongoing or completed antimicrobial treatment. This deterioration most commonly manifests more than 3 months after initiation of ART, so-called late IRIS or paradoxic IRIS and is hypothesized to result from an inflammatory reaction to nonviable pathogens. In the second scenario,

Positive Health Program at San Francisco General Hospital, University of California San Francisco, Building 80, Ward 84, 995 Potrero Avenue, San Francisco, CA 94110, USA
E-mail address: gbeatty@php.ucsf.edu

Emerg Med Clin N Am 28 (2010) 393–407
doi:10.1016/j.emc.2010.01.004   emed.theclinics.com
0733-8627/10/$ – see front matter © 2010 Elsevier Inc. All rights reserved.

immune reconstitution may unmask previously undiagnosed or occult infectious processes. This unmasking IRIS may produce symptoms that are not characteristic of the usual presentation of the infection, confounding diagnostic efforts. This presentation most commonly manifests within the first 3 months after initiation of ART, so-called early IRIS.

DEFINITION OF IRIS

Research into the incidence and spectrum of disorders of IRIS has been hampered by the lack of a consistent definition of the syndrome. A useful proposed definition of IRIS includes (1) symptoms occurring in a patient infected with HIV currently receiving ART, (2) a decrease in HIV-1 RNA levels from baseline and increase in CD4 cell count from baseline, (3) clinical symptoms consistent with an inflammatory process, and (4) a clinical course not consistent with the expected course of a previously diagnosed opportunistic infection, the expected course of a newly diagnosed opportunistic infection, or with drug toxicity (**Box 1**).[1]

INCIDENCE AND RISK FACTORS

IRIS occurs in 15% to 30% of all patients who initiate antiretroviral therapy, with a higher incidence in patients who have been diagnosed with an active opportunistic infection at the time of ART initiation.[1–4] Risk factors for the development of IRIS include a high baseline HIV viral load before initiation of ART, rapid decline in HIV viral load after initiation of ART, a lower baseline CD4 count before ART initiation, a high antigenic burden and disseminated (as opposed to localized) opportunistic infection, initiation of ART concomitant with or soon after initiation of treatment of an acute infection, and lack of exposure to ART before initiating the current regimen (**Box 2**). To date, age, gender, and type of antiretroviral regimen used have not been shown to consistently predict a patient's risk of IRIS.[2,4–8]

INFECTIONS ASSOCIATED WITH IRIS

A variety of fungal, parasitic, mycobacterial, and viral opportunistic infections are associated with manifestations of IRIS (**Tables 1** and **2**). Novel IRIS manifestations

---

Box 1
Definition of IRIS

- *Working definition of IRIS*
- Symptoms occurring in a patient who is HIV-positive currently receiving ART
- Immunologic response to antiretroviral therapy, as shown by:
  - Decrease in HIV-1 RNA levels from baseline
  - Increase in CD4 cell count from baseline
- Clinical symptoms consistent with an inflammatory process
- Clinical course *not* consistent with:
  - The expected course of a previously diagnosed opportunist infection
  - The expected course of a newly diagnosed opportunist infection
  - Drug toxicity

Box 2
Risk factors for IRIS
Lower baseline CD4 count and CD4% at initiation of ART
Rapid decline in HIV RNA on initiation of ART
ART-naive patient
Disseminated versus localized opportunistic infection
Initiation of ART soon after diagnosis/treatment of opportunistic infection
High baseline HIV RNA before initiation of ART

not previously reported may be encountered in the emergency care setting, and the following discussion does not comprise an exhaustive list of all pathogens reportedly associated with IRIS.

Fungal and Parasitic Infections

The most concerning manifestations of IRIS are those that occur in the closed space of the cranium. Approximately 5% to 8% of patients with AIDS not taking ART develop cryptococcal meningitis, and as many as 30% of these patients develop cryptococcal IRIS after starting ART (range 4%–66%).[7–10] The median time to development of symptoms after initiation of ART is approximately 30 to 45 days, with approximately 60% of cases occurring within the first month, although the symptoms may present as late as 10 to 12 months after treatment, and have been reported as far out as 3 years.[1,8,11–13] Manifestations of cryptococcal IRIS include recurrent meningitis, lymphadenitis, pneumonitis, and localized fungal abscess.[14] Because of the higher burden of cryptococcal disease in developing countries, cryptococcal IRIS contributes substantially to early morbidity and mortality in patients initiating ART in this setting. Specific risk factors for the development of cryptococcal IRIS that have been reported in some but not all studies include initiation of ART within 2 months of the treatment of *Cryptococcus* and high baseline cerebrospinal fluid (CSF) cryptococcal antigen titer. Severity of symptoms seems to be related to how long patients have received treatment of cryptococcal meningitis.[7,8,15] The most common presentation is that of an apparent relapse of previously treated meningitis in a patient newly treated with ART. On lumbar puncture, CSF opening pressure is typically high, and although cryptococcal antigen will be detected, CSF fungal cultures are negative. One retrospective study found that compared with classic forms of AIDS-related cryptococcal meningitis, patients with cryptococcal IRIS had significantly higher opening pressures, CSF white blood cell (WBC) counts (56 vs 12 cells/μL) and CD4 counts, and lower HIV viral loads.[7] Mortality from cryptococcal IRIS may be high, and the role of steroids in management remains unclear.

Table 1		
Types of infections associated with IRIS and typical time course of occurrence		
Pathogen Type	**Example**	**Typical Time Course**
Fungal	*Cryptococcus*	1 week to 12 months
Viral	Cytomegalovirus, herpes simplex virus	1 month to 3 years
Mycobacterial	*Mycobacterium avium* complex, tuberculosis	1–12 weeks
Autoimmune disease	Graves disease, sarcoid	1–3 years

Table 2
Common infections associated with IRIS and manifestations

Pathogen	IRIS Manifestation	Pathogen	IRIS Manifestation
Tuberculosis	Fever and weight loss New or worsening pulmonary infiltrates Pleural effusion Peritonitis Pericarditis Arthritis Steomyelitis Lymphadenitis Expansion of intracranial tuberculomas Hepatitis Skin or visceral abscess Hypercalcemia	Mycobacterium avium complex	Lymphadenitis Fever Soft tissue abscess Hepatosplenomegaly Paraspinal mass Abdominal pain Lymphadenopathy Pulmonary infiltrates Peritonitis Hypercalcemia Cytopenias
Cryptococcus neoformans	Recurrent headache Meningeal signs Lymphadenitis Cavitating pneumonia CNS cryptoccocoma	Hepatitis B	Increased transaminase levels Abdominal pain Tender hepatomegaly Nausea and vomiting Rapid progression of cirrhosis
Cytomegalovirus	Blurred vision Visual floaters Vitreitis Uveitis Retinitis Macular edema Blindness (late)	Progressive multifocal leukoencephalopathy (JC virus)	Worsening of neurocognitive and motor deficits
Pneumocystis jirovecci pneumonia	New cough Hypoxia Pneumonitis Respiratory failure after withdrawal of steroids	Herpes simplex virus	Genital ulceration
Varicella zoster virus	Zoster	Human herpes virus 8	New or worsening Kaposi sarcoma lesions

Pneumonia caused by *Pneumocystis jirovecci*, formerly *Pneumocystis carinii* (PCP), is one of the more common opportunistic infections in patients with advanced HIV disease. Worsening of active, treated PCP may occur within the first 2 to 3 weeks after initiation of ART, and less commonly as a later manifestation around 3 to 4 months after ART initiation.[16–18] Patients with PCP IRIS may present with worsening hypoxia, recrudescence of fever and pulmonary infiltrates on chest radiograph. This symptomology can be difficult to distinguish from PCP treatment failure. Patients with severe PCP (Pao_2 <70), those starting ART soon after initiation of PCP treatment, and those recently completing steroid therapy for PCP may be at higher risk.[16,19] Fatalities have been reported. Development of severe organizing pneumonia requiring mechanical ventilation shortly after cessation of antimicrobial and steroid therapy may also occur, a pattern that is highly unusual for treated PCP.[19]

IRIS associated with histoplasmosis is less common but has been reported from 3 weeks to 4 months after initiation of ART, and may present with pulmonary nodules and mediastinal lymphadenopathy. A hemophagocytic syndrome presenting with a fever, hepatosplenomegaly, pancytopenia, and disseminated intravascular coagulation (DIC) has been reported.[20]

Central nervous system (CNS) toxoplasmosis IRIS has been less thoroughly described although case reports exist. Clinical manifestations are those of toxoplasmic encephalitis, with fever, seizure, and/or focal neurologic deficit.[21]

Mycobacterial Infections

IRIS may occur in up to one-third of patients with disseminated *Mycobacterium avium* complex (MAC) following initiation of ART, and can affect multiple organ systems. MAC IRIS most commonly manifests as a suppurative painful lymphadenitis with fever, and can involve mediastinal, hilar, retroperitoneal, cervical, or intraabdominal nodes.[22,23] MAC IRIS has also been reported to involve the lungs, joints, skin, soft tissue, prostate, and brain.[24] In contrast to disseminated MAC disease of advanced AIDS, MAC IRIS lesions consist of well-organized granulomas, and significant hypercalcemia can occur and may be a presenting symptom. Onset of symptoms usually occurs within the first 12 weeks after initiation of ART but may be delayed by several months. Not uncommonly, MAC IRIS occurs in patients who are not known to have MAC at the time of ART initiation, thus unmasking the occult infection.[23,24]

Tuberculosis (TB) IRIS occurs in approximately 20% (range 8%–43%) of patients being treated for TB at the time of ART initiation.[6,25–27] As with other opportunistic infections, lower baseline CD4 count, high plasma viral load, and earlier start on ART relative to beginning anti-TB therapy are predictive of IRIS. Extrapulmonary or disseminated disease also portends higher risk.[28,29] Most cases of TB IRIS occur in patients initiating ART within 2 months of starting TB therapy.[30] Symptoms typically develop within 4 to 6 weeks after initiation of ART, with approximately 70% of cases presenting in the first 2 months.[28] Most common presentations include fever, cervical or intrathoracic lymphadenopathy (present in approximately 45% of cases), worsening of preexisting pulmonary infiltrates, or new infiltrates or pleural effusion on chest radiograph (24%), with or without respiratory symptoms.[24,31,32] Between 5% and 40% of cases involve intraabdominal manifestations.[6,28,32] CNS involvement, including tuberculosis abscesses and meningitis, occur in about 5% to 12% of cases and are of particular concern, given the attendant risk for neurologic deterioration.[33] Other manifestations of TB IRIS include visceral or cutaneous abscesses, arthritis, hepatitis, pericardial effusion, and osteomyelitis. Hypercalcemia has also been described, as has renal failure, orchitis, ocular involvement, and spontaneous splenic rupture.[34,35] Although it may be associated with substantial morbidity, TB IRIS is not often fatal.

Although corticosteroids are routinely used in the management of TB meningitis, their role in CNS TB IRIS remains unclear.[36]

Viral Infections

Some of the most clinically significant viral infections associated with IRIS include members of the herpes virus family: cytomegalovirus (CMV), herpes simplex virus (HSV), and varicella zoster virus (VZV). Three distinct ocular lesions associated with CMV IRIS have been described: retinitis, vitreitis, and uveitis. The first of these, CMV retinitis IRIS, is difficult to distinguish from active CMV retinitis. New retinal lesions may appear at the site of previously diagnosed retinitis within 2 months of initiation of ART. Unfortunately, IRD appears identical to active retinitis on fundoscopic examination, and IRIS is distinguished from active retinitis only by noting a gradual clearing of lesions in the absence of anti-CMV therapy in a patient who has recently started on ART.[37]

A more dramatic clinical presentation occurs in patients with CMV vitreitis, in which patients with preexisting diagnoses of CMV retinitis present with an acute onset of visual blurring 1 to 2 months after initiation of ART. Blurred vision is caused by infiltration of the vitreous humor with inflammatory cells, a self-limiting process that resolves in approximately 1 month without residual visual loss. The treatment is patient reassurance.[38]

In contrast, CMV uveitis usually results in some degree of permanent visual loss. Uveitis presents as painless visual loss in patients with a history of extensive retinitis relatively late after ART initiation, with a median time to onset of symptoms of 3 years. Restarting therapy for CMV or treating patients with steroids has not been shown to affect the course of uveitis.[37]

Antiretroviral therapy may increase the risk of herpes zoster by as much as 5-fold, and although most patients experience typical dermatomal distribution of new cutaneous lesions, more complicated presentations have been reported, including acute retinal necrosis, myelitis, mononeuritis, vasculopathy, and encephalitis.[11,39–42] IRIS associated with herpes zoster virus typically occurs as a late IRIS, after the first 3 months of ART.

As a general rule, cutaneous and visceral lesions of Kaposi sarcoma (KS) improve on initiation of ART. However, a minority of patients will experience worsening of preexisting lesions, typically within 8 weeks but possibly as late as 6 months after ART initiation.[43] The clinical course is typically that of a worsening of preexisting cutaneous lesions that resolve within a few months without specific therapy for KS. Reported predictors of developing KS-associated IRIS include presence of pretreatment KS, edema, anemia, and detectable KS-associated herpes virus DNA, as well as the common predictors of CD4 cell count increase and change in HIV viral load.[44,45] Patients with visceral involvement at the time of ART initiation are at higher risk of complications, and may experience exacerbation of pulmonary disease indistinguishable from pulmonary KS itself, which may be fatal.[46–48] A rapidly fatal course culminating in multiorgan system failure, a consumptive coagulopathy, and circulatory collapse has been reported.[49,50]

Progressive multifocal leukoencephalopathy (PML) is a demyelinating CNS disorder caused by reactivation of JC virus and is seen with advanced immunosuppression. Although not common (approximately 5% of patients with AIDS), PML has historically carried a dismal prognosis, with high morbidity and mortality and no effective specific treatment. Although prognosis is improved in patients initiating ART, symptoms may worsen in a subset of patients, consistent with IRIS. PML IRIS presents anywhere between 1 week and 6 months after initiation of ART and is characterized by contrast-enhancing lesions on neuroimaging and severe inflammatory and demyelin-ating lesions histopathologically.[51] The clinical course varies from mild self-limiting neurologic deficits, to severe irreversible neurologic deficits, to death. Patients in whom PML is unmasked by IRIS may have a somewhat milder course, whereas patients with preexisting diagnoses of PML tend to develop IRIS earlier, have more lesions on magnetic resonance imaging (MRI), and have shorter survival and higher mortality.[51] Steroids have been used in cases of severe neurologic symptoms but a consistent benefit of steroid therapy has not been demonstrated.

As many as one-third of patients with chronic hepatitis B initiating ART experience increases in hepatic transaminase levels, and the risk of an increased alanine amino-transferase (ALT) level is increased 2- to 8-fold in patients with HIV and hepatitis B coinfection compared with HIV alone.[52] Patients with preexisting increases in ALT level and those with higher hepatitis B virus (HBV) DNA levels seem to be at increased risk.[53] IRIS to hepatitis B may be exceedingly difficult to discern from hepatotoxicity of ART, inadequately treated hepatitis, inadvertent withdrawal of hepatitis B therapy, or development of hepatitis B antiviral resistance. However, in 1 study, 22% of patients positive for hepatitis B surface antigen developed transaminase flares in which pertur-bations of immune system cytokines were correlated with ALT, HBV viral load, HIV viral load, and CD4 cell count, supporting a role of IRIS in a large percentage of HIV/HBV coinfected patients with increased liver function tests after ART initiation.[53] Typically, an antiretroviral regimen in a patient with HIV and hepatitis B coinfection includes tenofovir and either emtricitabine or lamivudine, which have anti-HBV activity. Failure to include agents with activity against hepatitis B in an ART regimen may place patients at higher risk of hepatitis flare on immune restoration. IRIS associated with hepatitis B most commonly presents as asymptomatic increases in hepatic transam-inase levels in the first 3 to 5 months after initiation of ART, although it may progress to fulminant hepatic failure and death.[54]

AUTOIMMUNE DISEASE ASSOCIATED WITH IRIS
Graves Disease

Several different autoimmune processes have been described in patients initiating ART, although a clear association with IRIS has yet to be defined for many. It is widely accepted that Graves disease occurring after ART initiation is a manifestation of IRIS. This occurs late in the course of immune restoration, with a median time to onset after ART initiation of 21 months. In one study the median CD4 count before initiation of therapy in patients who developed Graves disease was 10 cells/mm^3, indicating severe immunodeficiency at the time of ART initiation in this population.[55–58]

Sarcoidosis

Immune reconstitution sarcoidosis has been reported in several patients receiving ART, and this granulomatous inflammation must be distinguished from IRIS associ-ated with mycobacterial pathogens. These lesions are histologically similar to sarcoid-osis occurring in patients with no HIV infection. This IRIS manifestation typically presents later, up to 3 years after initiation of ART.[59,60] Symptoms are similar to those found in sarcoidosis in patients without HIV, with prominent respiratory and constitu-tional symptoms, although extrapulmonary involvement is also common, including eye, skin, spleen, liver, heart, lymph node, CNS, and salivary gland disease. Hypercal-cemia has also been reported.[60–62]

Other autoimmune diseases reportedly associated with IRIS include systemic lupus erythematosus, polymyositis, and rheumatoid arthritis.

SYMPTOMATIC PRESENTATIONS

Active, untreated opportunistic infections must be considered in the differential diagnosis for any patient infected with HIV on ART presenting to an emergency department, informed by knowledge of the patient's CD4 count. Unfortunately, distinguishing between an active opportunistic complication of AIDS and a manifestation of IRIS can be challenging, and few clinical clues that assist in this distinction are readily available to the acute care provider (**Tables 3** and **4**). Whether to consider IRIS in the differential diagnosis of a patient depends first on the appropriate clinical scenario: are the symptoms occurring in a previously untreated patient who has commenced ART within the past few months and achieved a reduction in HIV viral load with an increase in CD4 count? Are they occurring in a patient currently being treated or recently completing treatment of an opportunistic infection?

Headache and Focal Neurologic Deficit

Patients presenting with headache and fever should prompt an investigation for possible IRIS to *Cryptococcus* or tuberculosis in the form of meningitis. The presence of focal neurologic deficits or seizures may reflect IRIS-associated cryptococcal or tuberculous abscess, PML IRIS, or less often, IRIS to toxoplasmosis. Distinguishing between active CNS infection and IRIS is important in these scenarios, as the use of steroid therapy may prove beneficial in the case of IRIS, but could be catastrophic in the case of active ongoing infection. In addition to the appropriate clinical setting, a higher CSF opening pressure and higher CSF WBC count might suggest cryptococcal IRIS rather than cryptococcal meningitis. In the case of cryptococcal and tuberculous disease, CSF culture negativity is expected in cases of IRIS but these results are not available to the clinician in a timely manner. In a patient with suspected PML, contrast enhancement on MRI is highly suggestive of IRIS rather than progression of PML. Other pathogens reported to cause IRIS in the brain include HSV, VZV, and parvovirus B19.

Pulmonary Symptoms

Presentations of cough, fever, hypoxia, and worsening pulmonary infiltrates in patients recently started on ART can indicate IRIS to tuberculosis, MAC, *Pneumocystis*, *Cryptococcus*, or Kaposi sarcoma. IRIS-associated sarcoidosis should also be considered. IRIS related to *Pneumocystis* and tuberculosis is likely to occur in patients with these preexisting diagnoses, whereas pulmonary involvement of MAC IRIS may be more likely to account for symptoms in a patient without a preexisting infectious diagnosis. Cryptococcal IRIS may cause diffuse infiltrates and nodules on chest radiograph. MAC IRIS more often presents with infiltrates, inflammatory masses, cavitary lesions, or endobronchial lesions. Tuberculosis IRIS presents as recrudescence of preexisting pulmonary infiltrates, new pulmonary infiltrates, or plural effusion, but endobronchial lesions are not common. The patient presenting with *Pneumocystis* IRIS is likely to have recently completed antimicrobial and steroid therapy for PCP and may have an organizing pneumonia or interstitial pneumonitis. Patients with pulmonary KS-associated IRIS commonly, although not always, have coexisting cutaneous KS lesions that have recently worsened.[32]

Febrile Syndromes

IRIS must also be considered in the differential diagnosis for patients who have recently started ART presenting with febrile syndromes for which infectious causes cannot be uncovered. Fever and constitutional symptoms can be caused by multiple

Table 3
Possible IRIS-associated processes in differential diagnosis of clinical presentations

IRIS Presentation	Associated Pathogens or Processes	IRIS Presentation	Associated Pathogens or Processes
Hypoxia, pulmonary infiltrates	Tuberculosis *Mycobacterium avium* complex *Pneumocystis* *Cryptococcus* Sarcoid	Hypercalcemia	Tuberculosis *Mycobacterium avium* complex Sarcoid *Cryptococcus*
Pleuritis, pericarditis	Tuberculosis	Headache, meningeal signs, focal neurologic deficits	Cryptococcal meningitis or abscess Tuberculosis Progressive multifocal leukoencephalopathy Toxoplasmosis
Fever and constitutional symptoms	Tuberculosis Cryptococcal disease *Mycobacterium avium* complex	Abdominal pain, hepatosplenomegaly	*Mycobacterium avium* complex Tuberculosis Viral hepatitis
Bone or joint disease	Tuberculosis Rheumatoid arthritis Lupus	Blurred vision, decreased visual acuity	Cytomegalovirus uveitis Vitreitis

Table 4
Characteristics that may help distinguish IRIS from active infectious disease for selected pathogens

Disease	IRIS[a]	Active Infectious Disease
Cryptococcus neoformans	High CSF WBC count High CSF opening pressure relative to active meningitis Negative CSF fungal culture	Lower CSF WBC count (often <20) and lower opening pressure relative to IRIS Positive CSF fungal culture
Progressive multifocal leukoencephalopathy	Contrast enhancement of lesions on MRI	Lack of contrast enhancement of lesions on MRI
Kaposi sarcoma	Worsening of preexisting cutaneous lesions	New cutaneous lesions
Cytomegalovirus	Retinitis in area of preexisting retinal lesion; presence of vitreitis or uveitis	Retinitis in new location; vitreitis and uveitis do not result from active cytomegalovirus disease in AIDS
Mycobacterium avium complex	Localized lymphadenitis Organized granulomas Hypercalcemia	Fever, weight loss, diarrhea Lymphadenitis and granulomatous formation not seen in active disease
Pneumocystis carinii	Organizing pneumonia after tapering steroids	Classic interstitial, ground glass pattern on chest radiograph Severe organizing pneumonia not typically seen

[a] Note that listed characteristics are inconsistently present in cases of IRIS.

IRIS-related pathogens, but in patients with no localizing symptoms particular consideration should be given to IRIS associated with MAC, tuberculosis, or *Cryptococcus*.

Dermatologic Manifestations

Dermatologic disease is extremely common in HIV infection and cutaneous IRIS manifestations account for approximately 50% to 75% of all IRIS events. A multitude of skin presentations have been reported, in addition to the characteristic violaceous nodular lesions of KS and KS IRIS. Some of the more common inflammatory eruptions attributed to IRIS include eosinophilic folliculitis, acne vulgaris, and demodex folliculitis. The lymphadenitis seen with tuberculosis and MAC IRIS may extend to overlying skin, and subcutaneous nodules related to unmasked atypical mycobacteria, tuberculosis, and sarcoid IRIS have been reported. Umbilicated papules may result from cryptococcal IRIS or from IRIS to molluscum contagiosum. Cutaneous abscesses can be caused by IRIS related to *Cryptococcus*, tuberculosis, or MAC. When herpes zoster occurs in the setting of IRIS the presentation is that of a typical dermatomal distribution. Cutaneous and anogenital warts associated with human papilloma virus may also worsen in the setting of immune reconstitution.[63]

Abdominal Pain and Hepatitis

Patients presenting with abdominal pain in the weeks and months following initiation of ART have a broad differential diagnosis, but manifestations of IRIS may include the intraabdominal lymphadenitis of MAC or tuberculosis, visceral KS, or hepatitis. Hepatic involvement of IRIS most often consists of increased transaminase levels noted on routine laboratory examination, but as described earlier, IRIS to hepatitis B may cause tender hepatomegaly and rarely fulminant hepatic failure. There is no consensus regarding a role of IRIS in chronic hepatitis C infection. The patient with hepatitis after initiation of ART poses a particular diagnostic dilemma.

MANAGEMENT

Although certain manifestations of IRIS cause mortality, patients with IRIS do not have a higher mortality compared with other patients infected with HIV on ART, and seem to have higher rates of eventual viral suppression and immune reconstitution than those without symptoms of IRIS.[3,64] Thus, development of IRIS is seldom, if ever, an indication for cessation of ART. Interruption of ART may place a patient at risk for additional opportunistic infections, and the IRIS may recur when ART is reintroduced. No randomized prospective trials have addressed the optimal management of patients with IRIS. In cases where IRIS represents unmasking of a previously undiagnosed opportunistic infection, specific antimicrobial therapy directed at the pathogen should be commenced immediately. In contrast, when IRIS occurs in response to pathogen for which the patient has already completed treatment, and an active infection has been ruled out, there is no evidence that retreatment or indefinite continuation of specific antimicrobial therapy is of benefit. Nonsteroidal antiinflammatory drugs (NSAIDS) are commonly used to decrease inflammation in patients with IRIS. Cryptococcal and tuberculosis-associated IRIS occurring in the CNS have the highest reported mortality. Outside the CNS, mycobacterial-associated IRIS may cause significant morbidity and increased rates of hospitalization, but seems to have a low mortality. Use of steroids for patients presenting with CNS manifestations is commonplace, although a mortality benefit has yet to be demonstrated.[33,65] The development of PCP IRIS after discontinuation of steroid therapy suggests a role for the reintroduction of steroids in these patients. In general, it is prudent to use NSAIDS for milder manifestations of IRIS and to treat with steroids in cases of widespread severe inflammation, hypercalcemia, CNS manifestations, or inflammation that threatens airway compromise. Prednisone or prednisolone is often dosed at 1 to 1.5 mg/kg/d and tapered over several weeks. Surgical drainage of necrotic mycobacterial lympadenitis or abscesses has been anecdotally reported to be of benefit. In patients with cryptococcal CNS IRIS, CSF drainage may be of benefit. Zoster occurring in HIV disease is typically treated with acyclovir, and there may also be clinical benefit of acyclovir in IRIS-associated zoster. In cases of ocular CMV IRIS, systemic or periocular steroid injections have been used, but a clear benefit has not been demonstrated, and these treatment decisions should be deferred to an ophthalmologist.[32,40,55,65]

SUMMARY

IRIS must be considered in the differential diagnosis for any patient infected with HIV who has begun ART in the preceding months. Distinguishing between manifestations of IRIS and active infection is of paramount importance and poses a diagnostic challenge to the provider in the acute care setting. Presentations of IRIS are often atypical for the precipitating pathogen, and novel presentations are likely. Of the diseases associated with IRIS, mycobacteria and cryptococcal infections are commonly encountered, as are dermatologic symptoms in general. The most clinically significant complications of IRIS are those involving the CNS, lungs, and eye, and in many of these scenarios systemic steroids may be of benefit. Management should rarely include interruption of ART, except possibly in severe, life-threatening complications. Prospective trials of steroids and other strategies in the management of IRIS are needed.

REFERENCES

1. Shelburne SA, Montes M, Hamill RJ. Immune reconstitution inflammatory syndrome: more answers, more questions. J Antimicrob Chemother 2006;57(2): 167–70.
2. French MA, Lenzo N, John M, et al. Immune restoration disease after the treatment of immunodeficient HIV-infected patients with highly active antiretroviral therapy. HIV Med 2000;1(2):107–15.
3. Shelburne SA, Visnegarwala F, Darcourt J, et al. Incidence and risk factors for immune reconstitution inflammatory syndrome during highly active antiretroviral therapy. AIDS 2005;19(4):399–406.
4. Ratnam I, Chiu C, Kandala NB, et al. Incidence and risk factors for immune reconstitution inflammatory syndrome in an ethnically diverse HIV type 1-infected cohort. Clin Infect Dis 2006;42(3):418–27.
5. Jevtovic DJ, Salemovic D, Ranin J, et al. The prevalence and risk of immune restoration disease in HIV-infected patients treated with highly active antiretroviral therapy. HIV Med 2005;6(2):140–3.
6. Lawn SD, Myer L, Bekker LG, et al. Tuberculosis-associated immune reconstitution disease: incidence, risk factors and impact in an antiretroviral treatment service in South Africa. AIDS 2007;21(3):335–41.
7. Shelburne SA 3rd, Darcourt J, White AC Jr, et al. The role of immune reconstitution inflammatory syndrome in AIDS-related *Cryptococcus neoformans* disease in the era of highly active antiretroviral therapy. Clin Infect Dis 2005;40(7):1049–52.
8. Lortholary O, Fontanet A, Memain N, et al. Incidence and risk factors of immune reconstitution inflammatory syndrome complicating HIV-associated cryptococcosis in France. AIDS 2005;19(10):1043–9.
9. Lawn SD, Bekker LG, Myer L, et al. Cryptococcocal immune reconstitution disease: a major cause of early mortality in a South African antiretroviral programme. AIDS 2005;19(17):2050–2.
10. Kambugu A, Meya DB, Rhein J, et al. Outcomes of cryptococcal meningitis in Uganda before and after the availability of highly active antiretroviral therapy. Clin Infect Dis 2008;46(11):1694–701.
11. French MA. HIV/AIDS: immune reconstitution inflammatory syndrome: a reappraisal. Clin Infect Dis 2009;48(1):101–7.
12. Bicanic T, Meintjes G, Rebe K, et al. Immune reconstitution inflammatory syndrome in HIV-associated cryptococcal meningitis: a prospective study. J Acquir Immune Defic Syndr 2009;51(2):130–4.
13. Sungkanuparph S, Jongwutiwes U, Kiertiburanakul S. Timing of cryptococcal immune reconstitution inflammatory syndrome after antiretroviral therapy in patients with AIDS and cryptococcal meningitis. J Acquir Immune Defic Syndr 2007;45(5):595–6.
14. Singh N, Perfect JR. Immune reconstitution syndrome associated with opportunistic mycoses. Lancet Infect Dis 2007;7(6):395–401.
15. Sungkanuparph S, Filler SG, Chetchotisakd P, et al. Cryptococcal immune reconstitution inflammatory syndrome after antiretroviral therapy in AIDS patients with

cryptococcal meningitis: a prospective multicenter study. Clin Infect Dis 2009; 49(6):931–4.

16. Wislez M, Bergot E, Antoine M, et al. Acute respiratory failure following HAART introduction in patients treated for *Pneumocystis carinii* pneumonia. Am J Respir Crit Care Med 2001;164(5):847–51.

17. Koval CE, Gigliotti F, Nevins D, et al. Immune reconstitution syndrome after successful treatment of *Pneumocystis carinii* pneumonia in a man with human immunodeficiency virus type 1 infection. Clin Infect Dis 2002;35(4):491–3.

18. Shelburne SA 3rd, Hamill RJ, Rodriguez-Barradas MC, et al. Immune reconstitution inflammatory syndrome: emergence of a unique syndrome during highly active antiretroviral therapy. Medicine (Baltimore) 2002;81(3):213–27.

19. Jagannathan P, Davis E, Jacobson M, et al. Life-threatening immune reconstitution inflammatory syndrome after *Pneumocystis* pneumonia: a cautionary case series. AIDS 2009;23(13):1794–6.

20. De Lavaissiere M, Manceron V, Bouree P, et al. Reconstitution inflammatory syndrome related to histoplasmosis, with a hemophagocytic syndrome in HIV infection. J Infect 2009;58(3):245–7.

21. Tremont-Lukats IW, Garciarena P, Juarbe R, et al. The immune inflammatory reconstitution syndrome and central nervous system toxoplasmosis. Ann Intern Med 2009;150(9):656–7.

22. Race EM, Adelson-Mitty J, Kriegel GR, et al. Focal mycobacterial lymphadenitis following initiation of protease-inhibitor therapy in patients with advanced HIV-1 disease. Lancet 1998;351(9098):252–5.

23. Phillips P, Bonner S, Gataric N, et al. Nontuberculous mycobacterial immune reconstitution syndrome in HIV-infected patients: spectrum of disease and long-term follow-up. Clin Infect Dis 2005;41(10):1483–97.

24. Lawn SD, Bekker LG, Miller RF. Immune reconstitution disease associated with mycobacterial infections in HIV-infected individuals receiving antiretrovirals. Lancet Infect Dis 2005;5(6):361–73.

25. Breton G, Duval X, Estellat C, et al. Determinants of immune reconstitution inflammatory syndrome in HIV type 1-infected patients with tuberculosis after initiation of antiretroviral therapy. Clin Infect Dis 2004;39(11):1709–12.

26. Kumarasamy N, Chaguturu S, Mayer KH, et al. Incidence of immune reconstitution syndrome in HIV/tuberculosis-coinfected patients after initiation of generic antiretroviral therapy in India. J Acquir Immune Defic Syndr 2004;37(5):1574–6.

27. Burman W, Weis S, Vernon A, et al. Frequency, severity and duration of immune reconstitution events in HIV-related tuberculosis. Int J Tuberc Lung Dis 2007; 11(12):1282–9.

28. Leone S, Nicastri E, Giglio S, et al. Immune reconstitution inflammatory syndrome associated with *Mycobacterium* tuberculosis infection: a systematic review. Int J Infect Dis August 3, 2009 [online].

29. Manabe YC, Campbell JD, Sydnor E, et al. Immune reconstitution inflammatory syndrome: risk factors and treatment implications. J Acquir Immune Defic Syndr 2007;46(4):456–62.

30. Navas E, Martin-Davila P, Moreno L, et al. Paradoxical reactions of tuberculosis in patients with the acquired immunodeficiency syndrome who are treated with highly active antiretroviral therapy. Arch Intern Med 2002;162(1):97–9.

31. French MA, Price P, Stone SF. Immune restoration disease after antiretroviral therapy. AIDS 2004;18(12):1615–27.

32. Crothers K, Huang L. Pulmonary complications of immune reconstitution inflammatory syndromes in HIV-infected patients. Respirology 2009;14(4):486–94.

33. Pepper DJ, Marais S, Maartens G, et al. Neurologic manifestations of paradoxical tuberculosis-associated immune reconstitution inflammatory syndrome: a case series. Clin Infect Dis 2009;48(11):e96–107.

34. Tsao YT, Wu YC, Yang CS, et al. Immune reconstitution associated hypercalcemia. Am J Emerg Med 2009;27(5):629, e1–3.

35. Weber E, Gunthard HF, Schertler T, et al. Spontaneous splenic rupture as manifestation of the immune reconstitution inflammatory syndrome in an HIV type 1 infected patient with tuberculosis. Infection 2009;37(2):163–5.

36. Olalla J, Pulido F, Rubio R, et al. Paradoxical responses in a cohort of HIV-1-infected patients with mycobacterial disease. Int J Tuberc Lung Dis 2002;6(1):71–5.

37. Nguyen QD, Kempen JH, Bolton SG, et al. Immune recovery uveitis in patients with AIDS and cytomegalovirus retinitis after highly active antiretroviral therapy. Am J Ophthalmol 2000;129(5):634–9.

38. Zegans ME, Walton RC, Holland GN, et al. Transient vitreous inflammatory reactions associated with combination antiretroviral therapy in patients with AIDS and cytomegalovirus retinitis. Am J Ophthalmol 1998;125(3):292–300.

39. Tsang CS, Samaranayake LP. Immune reconstitution inflammatory syndrome after highly active antiretroviral therapy: a review. Oral Dis 2009. [Epub ahead of print].

40. Martinez E, Gatell J, Moran Y, et al. High incidence of herpes zoster in patients with AIDS soon after therapy with protease inhibitors. Clin Infect Dis 1998;27(6):1510–3.

41. Domingo P, Torres OH, Ris J, et al. Herpes zoster as an immune reconstitution disease after initiation of combination antiretroviral therapy in patients with human immunodeficiency virus type-1 infection. Am J Med 2001;110(8):605–9.

42. Newsome SD, Nath A. Varicella-zoster virus vasculopathy and central nervous system immune reconstitution inflammatory syndrome with human immunodeficiency virus infection treated with steroids. J Neurovirol 2009;15(3):288–91.

43. Feller L, Lemmer J. Insights into pathogenic events of HIV-associated Kaposi sarcoma and immune reconstitution syndrome related Kaposi sarcoma. Infect Agent Cancer 2008;3:1.

44. Bower M, Nelson M, Young AM, et al. Immune reconstitution inflammatory syndrome associated with Kaposi's sarcoma. J Clin Oncol 2005;23(22):5224–8.

45. Letang E, Almeida JM, Miro JM, et al. Predictors of immune reconstitution inflammatory syndrome-associated with Kaposi sarcoma in Mozambique: a prospective study. J Acquir Immune Defic Syndr October 1, 2009 [online].

46. Connick E, Kane MA, White IE, et al. Immune reconstitution inflammatory syndrome associated with Kaposi sarcoma during potent antiretroviral therapy. Clin Infect Dis 2004;39(12):1852–5.

47. Godoy MC, Rouse H, Brown JA, et al. Imaging features of pulmonary Kaposi sarcoma-associated immune reconstitution syndrome. AJR Am J Roentgenol 2007;189(4):956–65.

48. Martin J, Laker M, Clutter D, et al. Kaposi's Sarcoma-associated immune reconstitution inflammatory syndrome in Africa: initial findings from a prospective evaluation. In 16th Conference on retroviruses and opportunistic infections. Montreal, Canada, February 8–11, 2009.

49. Nathan RV. Suspected immune reconstitution inflammatory syndrome associated with the proliferation of Kaposi's sarcoma during HAART. AIDS 2007;21(6):775.

50. Crane HM, Deubner H, Huang JC, et al. Fatal Kaposi's sarcoma-associated immune reconstitution following HAART initiation. Int J STD AIDS 2005;16(1): 80–3.
51. Tan K, Roda R, Ostrow L, et al. PML-IRIS in patients with HIV infection: clinical manifestations and treatment with steroids. Neurology 2009;72(17):1458–64.
52. Ofotokun I, Smithson SE, Lu C, et al. Liver enzymes elevation and immune reconstitution among treatment-naive HIV-infected patients instituting antiretroviral therapy. Am J Med Sci 2007;334(5):334–41.
53. Crane M, Oliver B, Matthews G, et al. Immunopathogenesis of hepatic flare in HIV/hepatitis B virus (HBV)-coinfected individuals after the initiation of HBV-active antiretroviral therapy. J Infect Dis 2009;199(7):974–81.
54. Thio CL, Locarnini S. Treatment of HIV/HBV coinfection: clinical and virologic issues. AIDS Rev 2007;9(1):40–53.
55. Elston JW, Thaker H. Immune reconstitution inflammatory syndrome. Int J STD AIDS 2009;20(4):221–4.
56. Crum NF, Ganesan A, Johns ST, et al. Graves disease: an increasingly recognized immune reconstitution syndrome. AIDS 2006;20(3):466–9.
57. Knysz B, Bolanowski M, Klimczak M, et al. Graves' disease as an immune reconstitution syndrome in an HIV-1-positive patient commencing effective antiretroviral therapy: case report and literature review. Viral Immunol 2006;19(1):102–7.
58. Vos F, Pieters G, Keuter M, et al. Graves' disease during immune reconstitution in HIV-infected patients treated with HAART. Scand J Infect Dis 2006;38(2):124–6.
59. Haramati LB, Lee G, Singh A, et al. Newly diagnosed pulmonary sarcoidosis in HIV-infected patients. Radiology 2001;218(1):242–6.
60. Foulon G, Wislez M, Naccache JM, et al. Sarcoidosis in HIV-infected patients in the era of highly active antiretroviral therapy. Clin Infect Dis 2004;38(3):418–25.
61. Trevenzoli M, Cattelan AM, Marino F, et al. Sarcoidosis and HIV infection: a case report and a review of the literature. Postgrad Med J 2003;79(935):535–8.
62. Ferrand RA, Cartledge JD, Connolly J, et al. Immune reconstitution sarcoidosis presenting with hypercalcaemia and renal failure in HIV infection. Int J STD AIDS 2007;18(2):138–9.
63. Huiras E, Preda V, Maurer T, et al. Cutaneous manifestations of immune reconstitution inflammatory syndrome. Curr Opin HIV AIDS 2008;3(4):453–60.
64. Zolopa A, Andersen J, Powderly W, et al. Early antiretroviral therapy reduces AIDS progression/death in individuals with acute opportunistic infections: a multicenter randomized strategy trial. PLoS One 2009;4(5):e5575.
65. Murdoch DM, Venter WD, Van Rie A, et al. Immune reconstitution inflammatory syndrome (IRIS): review of common infectious manifestations and treatment options. AIDS Res Ther 2007;4:9.

Metabolic and Hepatobiliary Side Effects of Antiretroviral Therapy (ART)

Daniel M. Lugassy, MD[a],*, Brenna M. Farmer, MD[b],
Lewis S. Nelson, MD[c]

KEYWORDS

- HAART • Hepatobiliary • Metabolic
- Adverse drug events • Side effects

Highly active antiretroviral therapy (HAART), introduced in 1996, refers to the combination of 3 to 4 antiretroviral drugs used to prevent the progression of disease in patients infected by human immunodeficiency virus (HIV). Previously used monotherapy to treat HIV led to a high level of resistance, and was inferior to regimens that include 3 or more drugs.[1] Several different classes of drugs are used in HAART; the earliest included nucleoside reverse transcriptase inhibitors (NRTI), non-nucleoside reverse transcriptase inhibitors (NNRTI), and protease inhibitors (PI). Recently, additional classes have emerged which include fusion inhibitors, chemokine receptor inhibitors, and integrase inhibitors. It was initially perceived that this combination of antiretroviral therapy (ART) would be a cure for HIV, as it often produced remarkable recovery, and arrested the progression of the disease. However, these findings were spurious and HIV is now considered a chronic disease that can be managed medically. A plethora of literature shows that ART has considerably decreased morbidity and mortality from infectious complications of HIV.[2,3] Life expectancy of young patients infected with HIV was 9.1 years in the pre-HAART era of the early 1990s, but now has increased to 23 to 35 years.[1]

Although the prevalence of opportunistic infections, AIDS-related illnesses, and complications have declined dramatically, it seems that patients infected with HIV on ART are now suffering from more HIV-related chronic illnesses including hepatic,

[a] New York City Poison Control Center, New York University School of Medicine, 455 First Avenue, Room 123, New York, NY 10016, USA
[b] Division of Emergency Medicine, Weill-Cornell Medical College, New York Presbyterian Hospital, 525 East 68th Street, M-130, New York, NY 10065, USA
[c] Department of Emergency Medicine, New York City Poison Control Center, New York University School of Medicine, 455 First Avenue, Room 123, New York, NY 10016, USA
* Corresponding author.
E-mail address: daniel.lugassy@nyumc.org

Emerg Med Clin N Am 28 (2010) 409–419
doi:10.1016/j.emc.2010.01.011
0733-8627/10/$ – see front matter © 2010 Elsevier Inc. All rights reserved.

cardiovascular, and pulmonary diseases.[4-6] The increased use of ART has been associated with the development of these chronic illnesses and adverse drug events.[3,5] It is important for the emergency physician to appreciate this phenomenon, as it has changed the traditional diagnoses of patients with HIV presenting to the emergency department (ED).[5] In 1 study the most prevalent diagnosis of patients with HIV discharged from the ED was ill-defined symptoms/signs.[7] There was no follow-up in this study, but some of these patients may have had unrecognized complications from ART.[4,8]

Although ART for HIV has been in use since 1987, the initiation of HAART has produced an increase in adverse drug reactions.[2,3] This is a new challenge as many of the adverse drug reactions attributable to ART may be indistinguishable from non–drug-related illnesses.[9] The emergency physician must be aware of the potential complications of ART as affected patients may present with nonspecific symptoms. The focus of this article is the metabolic and hepatobiliary adverse effects of ART. Complications are presented based on clinical effects rather than drug class. This is more practical for several reasons; first there are almost 30 different medications within the category of ART today and many medications have several names or abbreviations.[8] Several ART drugs have been combined into single pill regimens, creating another potential area of confusion. Patients on ART may not always know, remember, or be able to communicate their exact regimen. Several adverse effects overlap drug classes and it is more important to recognize and manage potential complications than to focus narrowly on adverse events known to occur from a given class. **Table 1** provides a quick reference to the drugs found in each class of ART and associated metabolic and hepatobiliary complications.

PHARMACOLOGY OF ART

The abbreviation NRTI refers to either nucleoside reverse transcriptase inhibitors or nucleotide reverse transcriptase inhibitors. Both have essentially the same mechanism of action; they are analogues of native deoxynucleotides, such as thymidine, guanosine, or uridine. The only difference between these 2 classes is that nucleosides need to be phosphorylated once they enter the cell. Their structure allows them to be incorporated into the growing viral DNA strand in place of their analogous nucleotide, acting as a competitive inhibitor of HIV-1 reverse transcriptase. This incorporation results in the premature termination of the growing viral DNA strand because they lack an essential hydroxyl group needed to create the proper bond linking the next nucleotide. NRTIs are the cornerstone of ART. NNRTIs are noncompetitive inhibitors of HIV-1 reverse transcriptase, binding to a different site than NRTIs. This mechanism allows them to be used synergistically with NRTIs to decrease viral DNA reverse transcription. Protease inhibitors (PIs) prevent posttranslational enzyme activity in the final steps of HIV viral protein processing rendering them immature and noninfectious.

Newer drugs have emerged and have become incorporated into ART. Entry (fusion) inhibitors interfere with the complex binding and fusion of the HIV virus into the host cell. Chemokine coreceptor antagonists, considered by some to be a subclass of entry inhibitors, specifically arrest the entry of the HIV into the host cell by blocking receptors on the surface that are required for binding. Integrase inhibitors are able to block the action of the viral enzyme integrase that is responsible for the critical step of inserting the viral DNA into the host genome. These medications are relatively new and, although hepatotoxicity is a recognized adverse drug reaction (ADR), there is less known about the other possible adverse effects of these medications.

Table 1 Antiretroviral drugs used in ART, and associated metabolic and hepatobiliary adverse effects	
Medication Class	**Associated Adverse Effects**
NRTI (nucleoside/nucleotide reverse transcriptase inhibitors)	
Abacavir (Ziagen, ABC) Didanosine (Videx, ddI) Emtricitabine (Emtriva, FTC) Lamivudine (Epivir, 3TC) Stavudine (Zerit, d4T) Tenofovir (Viread, TDF) Zalcitabine (Hivid, ddC) Zidovudine (Retrovir, AZT, ZDV)	Hepatotoxicity Hepatic steatosis Pancreatitis Hypersensitivity syndrome Lactic acidosis
NNRTI (non-nucleoside reverse transcriptase inhibitors)	
Delavirdine (Rescriptor, DLV) Efavirenz (Sustiva, Stocrin, EFV) Etravirine (Intelence, TMC 125) Nevirapine (Viramune, NVP)	Hepatotoxicity Hepatic necrosis Hypersensitivity syndrome
Protease inhibitors	
Amprenavir (Agenerase, APV) Atazanavir (Reyataz, ATV) Darunavir (Prezista, DRV, TMC 114) Fosamprenavir (Lexiva, Telzir, FPV) Indinavir (Crixivan, IDV) Lopinavir/ritonavir (Kaletra) Nelfinavir (Viracept, NFV) Ritonavir (Norvir, RTV) Saquinavir (Invirase, SQV) Tipranavir (Aptivus, TPV)	Hepatotoxicity Hyperbilirubinemia Pancreatitis Dyslipidemia Hyperglycemia/insulin resistance Lipodystrophy
Entry (fusion) inhibitors	
Enfuvirtide (Fuzeon, ENF, T-20)	Hepatotoxicity Hypertriglyceridemia Hypersensitivity syndrome
Chemokine coreceptor antagonists	
Maraviroc (Selzentry, Celsentri, MVC)	Hepatotoxicity Lipodystrophy Hypersensitivity syndrome
Chemokine coreceptor antagonists	
Raltegravir (Isentress, RAL)	Hepatotoxicity Hypersensitivity syndrome

The latest recommended starting HAART regimens for patients who are naive to antiretroviral treatment are 1 of the following 2 combinations: 1 NNRTI + 2 NRTIs, or 2 NRTIs + 1 PI.[4] Each class has many different options and practitioners take several factors into consideration when choosing specific drugs in each class such as toxicities, pill burden, dosing frequency, and drug-drug interactions.

HEPATOBILIARY COMPLICATIONS

It is often difficult to determine whether hepatic injury is a direct medication side effect, drug-drug interaction, or unrelated to medications. Hepatic injury from ART may result in long-term liver damage with jaundice, cirrhosis, and fulminant hepatic failure.[10] Liver toxicity in HIV-infected patients increases health care costs as a result of prolonged hospital stays from ART associated toxicity.[9] Life-threatening events related to hepatic damage occur in about 2.6 per 100 person-years on ART.[8] Most effects are not life threatening but some patients who initially have benign presentations can progress to severe complications. Most hepatobiliary complications resolve with cessation of the inciting drug. Meticulous care must be taken to assess whether stopping part or all of the ART is needed. Patients who miss only a few doses of 1 or more of their medications even for a short period of time may develop viral resistance.[4,11]

Almost all antiretroviral drugs have been associated with hepatotoxicity as most of them are metabolized by the liver and the cytochrome P450 enzyme system.[4,8,10,11] Drug-induced hepatic injury may fall into 3 categories: hepatocellular, cholestatic, and a combination of the 2. Hepatocellular injury is direct hepatocyte damage that is often reflected by an elevation in transaminases.[8] Cholestatic injury occurs from blockage or damage to the biliary tree and is often reflected by elevations in bilirubin, γ-glutamyl transferase, and alkaline phosphatase.[8]

Once hepatic injury is suspected, the first step in the ED is to establish that the patient does not have signs or laboratory abnormalities consistent with hepatic compromise, such as ascites, hyperbilirubinemia, coagulopathy, or encephalopathy.[11] When evaluating a patient in the ED it is probably safe to hold their ART while determining their disposition. Ultrasound and computed tomography (CT) may show signs of hepatic abnormalities, but do not differentiate drug-related from non–drug-related injury.[11] Even a liver biopsy may be not be sufficient to distinguish a drug reaction from another medical cause.[8] Although there is no clear evidence or consensus to date on which patients require admission, those who are symptomatic warrant observation or close follow-up within 12 to 24 hours to prevent the progression of 1 of the adverse events reviewed later in this article.

ARTs are believed to cause hepatotoxicity via 4 mechanisms: direct drug toxicity, hypersensitivity reactions, mitochondrial toxicity, and immune reconstitution.[8,10] The discussion in this article concentrates on the first 3 mechanisms and how each pertains to the hepatobiliary adverse effects. The fourth, immune reconstitution, is a response to dormant infections, including hepatitis, with the initiation of ART and is covered in another article.

Hepatitis and Increased Transaminase Levels

Hepatotoxicity resulting in hepatocellular damage may occur as a direct effect of the parent drug or via accumulation of toxic metabolites created via the cytochrome P450 system in the liver. Various genetic changes, drug interactions, and gene polymorphisms in the P450 system may significantly alter a patient's susceptibility to damage from a drug.[10] The most commonly used markers to screen for hepatocellular injury are aspartate aminotransferase (AST) and alanine aminotransferase (ALT). Both of these markers are sensitive for injury but have poor specificity and prognostic value. Hepatic injury is often defined as increases in AST/ALT levels that are 3 to 5 times more than the upper limits of normal or the patient's baseline values before initiation of ART. About 5% to 10% of patients have increased liver enzyme levels after the initiation of ART, with 6% to 18% progressing to severe hepatotoxicity.[8,11] Most patients have mild increases in their AST/ALT levels within the first few months of ART, which may occur with or without symptoms.[12] All drug classes of ART have the potential to cause severe liver injury progressing to fulminant hepatic failure.[12] Although the injury may be caused by ART, the differential diagnosis of such increases is vast, including acute or chronic viral hepatitis (hepatitis A, B, C or D, cytomegalovirus, Epstein-Barr virus), ethanol or substance abuse, systemic or opportunistic infections, nonalcoholic steatosis, and malignancies.[11,13]

In the ED, patients with hepatocellular damage warrant evaluation for drug-induced, viral-associated, or other causes of hepatotoxicity.[11] It is sensible to obtain a serum acetaminophen concentration given that this is one of the most common causes of fulminant hepatic failure worldwide. Patients infected with HIV with clinical signs of hepatitis, such as fatigue, nausea, vomiting, and right upper quadrant abdominal pain and tenderness should be admitted for further evaluation and treatment. Consideration must given to stopping 1 or more of the drugs in the patient's ART drug regimen if the symptoms are significant.[8] There are no clear guidelines on how to manage isolated transaminase increases that are mild and do not concurrently exist with signs of other organ dysfunction or hepatic compromise. These patients should have close follow-up and clear instructions to return to the ED if symptoms worsen.

Increase in Bilirubin Level

The PIs have been associated with hyperbilirubinemia. Atazanavir and indinivir cause isolated hyperbilirubinemia without increase in transaminase levels. About 40% of individuals receiving atazanavir develop a significant increase in their total bilirubin level, 5% of patients develop jaundice, although none of them develop clinically significant hepatotoxicity.[14] This increase in total bilirubin level may be caused by a similar mechanism as Gilbert syndrome involving inhibition of UGT1A1 (UDP glucuronosyl transferase), an enzyme required for conjugation of bilirubin.[15] Indinivir causes unconjugated hyperbilirubinemia in 10% of patients, also without any other evidence of hepatotoxicity. Similar to atazanivir, the mechanism of indinavir-related hyperbilirubinemia is also analogous to Gilbert syndrome and related to specific haplotypes of UDP glucuronosyl transferase.[16,17] Jaundice may occur without actual hepatic damage and is reversible if the drug is discontinued, but this may not be needed if the patient is asymptomatic.[8] Hyperbilirubinemia from PIs are not associated with hepatotoxicity and should not be confused with posthepatic cholestasis, which presents as a delayed increase in bilirubin level seen after hepatocellular injury caused by regeneration of hepatocytes reconnecting with the biliary tree.[12]

Hypersensitivity Syndrome

Hypersensitivity syndrome is a life-threatening syndrome that is caused by an immune reaction to either the parent drug or a metabolite.[10] The classic and probably most well-recognized cause is abacavir, an NRTI, but it also occurs with agents from other ART classes (see **Table 1**). The presence of the drug evokes an immune-mediated response that can affect the liver as well as other organs, such as the skin, lungs, kidney, and heart. It most often occurs within the first few days of initiating therapy, but may occur as late as 8 weeks. Appearing suddenly, patients reliably note an exacerbation and progression of symptoms with each successive dose. The most common symptoms are fever, rash, nausea, and vomiting. In abacavir hypersensitivity, 80% of patients have a fever, and 70% have a rash.[10] Patients may also exhibit myalgias, headache, diarrhea, pruritis, lymphadenopathy, mucocutaneous involvement, hypotension, and respiratory symptoms such as cough, dyspnea, or pharyngitis.[8,10,18] Hypersensitivity is usually associated with increased transaminase levels in addition to the presence of other laboratory abnormalities such as leukopenia, thrombocytopenia, increased serum creatinine level, increased creatine phosphokinase level, and eosinophilia.[12] It is critical to have a high suspicion for the presence of this syndrome, as it may progress rapidly to multisystem organ failure even with aggressive and appropriate supportive care.[12]

Although it may be difficult to distinguish hypersensitivity from infectious or other underlying disorders, it has been recommended that all ART be held if the patient has 2 or more of the following symptoms: fever, rash, gastrointestinal symptoms, constitutional symptoms, and respiratory symptoms. In patients with mild symptoms or less than 2 of these symptoms, patients may continue to take their medications with close observation. Consultation with either the admitting physician or the patient's HIV primary care provider is suggested. The vague nature of these symptoms may result in over diagnosis of hypersensitivity, unnecessarily precluding the use of the suspected drug in the future.

Cessation of the offending agent is currently the only effective treatment, with resolution of most symptoms within 48 to 72 hours. Corticosteroids have failed to show a benefit in prophylaxis and therapy. Communication with the patient and any physician who cares for a patient with a suspected hypersensitivity reaction is critical.[12] Be aware that several medications combine abacavir with other drugs under completely different names and patients may not appreciate this potential hazard of unintended rechallenge.

Genetics may play a role in the occurrence and severity of adverse drug events. In the case of abacavir, there has been an association between developing hypersensitivity and several alleles including a strong link with HLA-B*5701. Currently genetic prescreening for HLA-B*5701 is recommended before initiation of abacavir for all patients.[10,19]

Hepatic Steatosis

Mitochondrial damage is believed to be a prominent cause of hepatic steatosis. The NRTIs can reduce the replication of mitochondrial DNA (mtDNA) in a manner similar to their effects on the HIV DNA replication.[13,20] mtDNA produces several of the subunits that form the electron transport chain found on the inner membranes of mitochondria. Without efficient functioning of this pathway, oxidative phosphorylation is impaired, which leads to an accumulation of fatty acids and other precursors in the cell. This results in hepatic steatosis, also known as nonalcoholic fatty liver disease.[20] It has also been associated with several metabolic and endocrine disorders, including diabetes, cirrhosis, metabolic syndrome, and cardiovascular disease. Hepatic steatosis may have a relatively benign or even asymptomatic presentation and may also mimic other diseases such as alcohol-induced liver injury, pregnancy steatosis, and Reye syndrome.[11] Patients may present with mild symptoms suggestive of hepatitis, such as abdominal pain, nausea, and vomiting. Hepatic steatosis rarely progresses to cause hepatic compromise.[21]

Lactic Acidosis

One of the most severe complications recognized as a risk of ART is the development of symptomatic hyperlactatemia with metabolic acidosis.[22] Lactate, under aerobic conditions, is oxidized to pyruvate using NAD+ and the enzymatic activity of lactate dehydrogenase. The mitochondrial toxicity responsible for causing hepatic steatosis may also cause this disorder, which seems to be exclusive to NRTIs.[20] Disruption of oxidative phosphorylation prevents aerobic energy production and eliminates lactate clearance.[13,23]

Several recognized criteria have been used to define this complication. Patients may have a lactic acidemia which refers to any increase in lactate more than normal without laboratory evidence of acidosis. Lactate increases are classified as mild (2–5 mmol/L), moderate (5–10 mmol/L), and severe (>10 mmol/L). A patient is considered to have lactic acidosis if their pH is less than 7.3 and bicarbonate less than 20 mEq/L with any abnormal increase in serum lactate level.[23] Patients may present with nonspecific symptoms such as fatigue, general malaise, nausea, vomiting, abdominal pain, hepatotoxicity, tender hepatomegaly, peripheral edema, and ascites.[23] Severe cases may progress rapidly to cardiomyopathy, encephalopathy, peripheral neuropathy, pancreatitis, panyctopenia, fulminant hepatic failure, and cardiopulmonary shock.[8,20,23] Severe symptoms occur in up to 25.2 of every 1000 person-years of ART, with a mortality of 30% to 60%.[23]

In patients with no symptoms, a screening lactate is not indicated.[24] Because of the vague nature and poor correlation of symptoms to the degree of increase in lactate or acidosis, patients on ARTs who present to the ED with any systemic complaints should be screened with a venous lactate, pH, bicarbonate level, and hepatic function panel.[24] Lactic acidosis may develop within months to years after the initiation of ART (specifically an NRTI). Factors that increase the risk for this adverse event include NRTI use greater than 6 months, pregnancy, female sex, age greater than 40 years, lower CD4 count, concurrent use of stavudine and didanosine, use of hydroxyurea or ribavirin with didanosine, obesity, and an increased body mass index (calculated as weight in kilograms divided by the square of height in meters).[12,23,25]

Managing these patients in the ED varies based on the serum lactate concentrations, symptoms, and suspicion for other causes of increased lactate. Patients with moderate to severe increases in serum lactate level, with an acidosis, or who are symptomatic should have their NRTI discontinued immediately.[20] Any concurrent condition such as metabolic acidosis, renal failure, or other organ dysfunction should be addressed as usual. No systematic trials or clear consensus exists on how to treat these patients beyond drug discontinuation and supportive care. Adjunctive therapies used in the treatment of other causes of lactic acidosis, such as sodium bicarbonate therapy, mechanical ventilation, and hemodialysis with bicarbonate buffer have been used with some success, but none have proved to be routinely beneficial. Because of the proposed mechanism of mitochondrial dysfunction, several cofactors have also been used with varying success, including thiamine, riboflavin, L-carnitine, and coenzyme Q.[12,23] Although they are all relatively benign therapies, they also have yet to show a clear benefit.

Pancreatitis

Pancreatitis is a common adverse event attributable to ART. Advanced HIV disease alone is associated with an increased incidence of pancreatitis, but NRTI use is independently linked to this complication.[26] Patients present with complaints similar to patients with non-ART causes of pancreatitis, including nausea, abdominal pain, vomiting, and fever.[27,28] The incidence of pancreatitis in patients on didanosine (NRTI) ranges from 1% to 7%, with a 6% mortality if it occurs.[29] This complication occurs most often 2 to 5 months after the initiation of ART. The concurrent use of didanosine (NRTI) with hydroxyurea should be avoided as it dangerously multiplies the risk of pancreatitis 4-fold. Stavudine, an NRTI, seems to incur a greater risk of lactic acidosis compared with other NRTIs.[25] Other known risk factors are a CD4 count less than 200 cells/mm^3, age greater than 37 years old, increased baseline amylase, and female gender.[27,30,31]

The mechanism of pancreatic toxicity may be related to the mitochondrial toxicity of NRTIs, as discussed earlier for lactic acidosis and hepatic steatosis. PIs often induce hyperlipidemia, a known cause of pancreatitis. Patients who have clinical symptoms consistent with pancreatitis while on ART should have serum lipase concentrations measured. Increase in pancreatic enzymes 2 to 3 times more than normal with clinical symptoms confirms this diagnosis. There is no evidence to support the screening of pancreatic enzymes in patients who are asymptomatic.

Patients who develop pancreatitis while on ART are treated by discontinuing the drug, and providing supportive care including bowel rest, analgesics, intravenous fluid therapy, and parental nutrition if needed. In addition, controlling hyperlipidemia in patients on PIs may prevent as well as treat pancreatitis.

METABOLIC COMPLICATIONS

The metabolic complications associated with ARTs may indirectly increase the risk of several acute life-threatening conditions such as diabetic ketoacidosis and myocardial infarction. The treatment of these complications does not differ from the standard therapy provided for patients not infected with HIV, but physicians should recognize ART as a nontraditional risk factor for these medical diseases.

Hyperglycemia/Insulin Resistance

Before the development of ARTs, there was no recognized association between HIV infection and alterations in glucose metabolism. PIs have been found to cause hyperglycemia caused by peripheral insulin resistance resulting in diabetes mellitus in some patients and worsening diabetes in patients with preexisting disease.[32–35] Patients may develop hyperglycemia or present with diabetic ketoacidosis, generally within 11 weeks of starting a PI.[36] Specifically, indinivir is associated with hyperglycemia and insulin resistance in healthy volunteers without HIV infection, even after only 1 dose.[37] The mechanism of insulin resistance is likely related to the inhibition of the GLUT-4 transporter found in pancreatic, fat, skeletal, and cardiac muscles cells.[20,38] Another possible mechanism may be an increase in pancreatic β-islet cell apoptosis.[39]

Management is the same as that provided to patients without HIV, including the use of oral antidiabetic or hypoglycemic agents, the use of insulin, and close monitoring of serum glucose levels.[40] In the ED, patients on PIs should have their serum glucose levels checked. If increased, screening for diabetic ketoacidosis should include the assessment of serum pH, bicarbonate level, anion gap, and serum and/or urine ketones, as appropriate.

Dyslipidemia

Dyslipidemia, resulting in hypercholesterolemia, hypertriglyceridemia, increased low-density lipoproteins, and reduced high-density lipoproteins is another metabolic complication of ART specifically associated with PIs. These metabolic changes have been seen as early as a few weeks after initiation of ART. Enfuvirtide, a fusion inhibitor, increased triglycerides in 8.9% of patients in clinical trials.[41] Approximately 50% of patients after 1 year on ART have newly diagnosed hyperlipidemia.[20]

There are several mechanisms believed to cause the dyslipidemia associated with ARTs, each mediated by alterations in different receptors and enzymes.[20] Ultimately they result in increased lipoprotein synthesis and impaired lipoprotein clearance.[42]

Initially, patients on ART were not found to have an increased risk of cardiovascular events, but recent studies show that increased lipid panels and the risk of cardiovascular disease increases with each year that a patient takes a PI.[43] Therefore, in addition to traditional risk factors such as smoking and hypertension, it seems that ART use should also be considered a cardiovascular risk factor.

Lipodystrophy/Fat Redistribution Syndrome

For years, generalized wasting was commonly seen as a complication of HIV from a loss of muscle mass.[20] Lipodystrophy, or fat redistribution syndrome, results from a combination of lipohypertrophy and lipoatrophy in patients on PIs and NRTIs.[44]

Increased fat accumulation may result in a buffalo hump, truncal obesity, and breast enlargement. Concurrently, there may be loss of fat in the subcutaneous tissues of the face, arms, and legs, leading to an altered body habitus.[20] The overall result is often an appearance of truncal obesity with peripheral wasting. The prevalence of this ill-defined condition is wide, ranging from 10% to 64% at 1 year and as high as 83% when approaching 2 years on ART.[20]

The mechanism of lipodystrophy is unclear. Patients may be managed with diet and exercise, but this may only exacerbate peripheral wasting. Although many of these changes seem Cushingoid, they have not been associated with changes in cortisol levels. This syndrome does not seem to be an acute concern to emergency physicians, but it may represent an increased risk for the other metabolic adverse effects of ART.

ADVERSE EFFECTS OF ART IN OVERDOSE AND POSTEXPOSURE PROPHYLAXIS

There is limited experience with intentional overdose of ARTs, but it seems that there may be no additional risks associated with an overdose of these medications outside of the already recognized adverse effects. Seizures are reported from zidovudine (NRTI).[45] In patients who are naive to these drugs it would seem extremely unlikely that metabolic complications would occur following a single acute ingestion, but many of the hepatobiliary complications have occurred after only a few doses. Patients who overdose on these medications may be on them chronically, so the same metabolic and hepatobiliary complications discussed earlier should be considered. The most concerning acute ADR would be a hypersensitivity syndrome.

Another population to consider at risk for complications of ARTs is patients with exposures to HIV who require postexposure HIV prophylaxis (PEP). The latest PEP recommendations are to prescribe 2 to 4 agents consisting of combinations of NRTIs and PIs.[12] The duration of therapy is often suggested to be at least 4 weeks. This is a significant exposure given that almost all of the metabolic and hepatobiliary complications have been known to occur within the first 4 weeks of therapy.[8] Lactic acidosis has been documented in patients on PEP therapy.[30] It is recommended that nevirapine not be given for PEP because of cases of hypersensitivity syndrome, fulminant hepatic failure, and severe hepatotoxicity with the use of this drug in several otherwise healthy patients.[12]

REFERENCES

1. Lima V, Hogg R, Harrigan PR, et al. Continued improvement in survival among HIV-infected individuals with newer forms of highly active antiretroviral therapy. AIDS 2007;21(6):685–92.
2. Pulvirenti J. Inpatient care of the HIV infected patient in the highly active antiretroviral therapy (HAART) era. Curr HIV Res 2005;3(2):133–45.
3. Pulvirenti J, Muppidi U, Glowacki R, et al. Changes in HIV-related hospitalizations during the HAART era in an inner-city hospital. AIDS Read 2007;17(8):390–4, 397.
4. Venkat A, Piontkowsky DM, Cooney RR, et al. Care of the HIV-positive patient in the emergency department in the era of highly active antiretroviral therapy. Ann Emerg Med 2008;52(3):274–85.
5. Llibre JM, Falco V, Tural C, et al. The changing face of HIV/AIDS in treated patients. Curr HIV Res 2009;7(4):365–77.
6. Palella F, Baker R, Moorman A, et al. Mortality in the highly active antiretroviral therapy era: changing causes of death and disease in the HIV outpatient study. J Acquir Immune Defic Syndr 2006;43(1):27–34.

7. Venkat A, Shippert B, Hanneman D, et al. Emergency department utilization by HIV-positive adults in the HAART era. Int J Emerg Med 2008;1(4):287–96.
8. Puoti M, Nasta P, Gatti F, et al. HIV-related liver disease: ARV drugs, coinfection, and other risk factors. J Int Assoc Physicians AIDS Care 2009;8(1):30–42.
9. Nunez M, Martn-Carbonero L, Moreno V, et al. Impact of antiretroviral treatment-related toxicities on hospital admissions in HIV-infected patients. AIDS Res Hum Retroviruses 2006;22(9):825–9.
10. Hughes CA, Foisy MM, Dewhurst N, et al. Abacavir hypersensitivity reaction: an update. Ann Pharmacother 2008;42(3):387–96.
11. Kottilil S, Polis M, Kovacs J. HIV infection, hepatitis C infection, and HAART: hard clinical choices. JAMA 2004;292(2):243–50.
12. Nunez M, Soriano V. Hepatotoxicity of antiretrovirals: incidence, mechanisms and management. Drug Saf 2005;28(1):53–66.
13. Cote HC, Brumme ZL, Craib KJ, et al. Changes in mitochondrial DNA as a marker of nucleoside toxicity in HIV-infected patients. N Engl J Med 2002;346(11):811–20.
14. Goldsmith DR, Perry CM. Atazanavir. Drugs 2003;63(16):1679–93 [discussion: 1694–5].
15. Havlir DV, O'Marro SD. Atazanavir: new option for treatment of HIV infection. Clin Infect Dis 2004;38(11):1599–604.
16. Plosker GL, Noble S. Indinavir: a review of its use in the management of HIV infection. Drugs 1999;58(6):1165–203.
17. Lankisch TO, Behrens G, Ehmer U, et al. Gilbert's syndrome and hyperbilirubinemia in protease inhibitor therapy–an extended haplotype of genetic variants increases risk in indinavir treatment. J Hepatol 2009;50(5):1010–8.
18. Bonfanti P, Capetti A, Riva P, et al. Hypersensitivity reactions during antiretroviral regimens with protease inhibitors. AIDS 1997;11(10):1301–2.
19. Sheffield LJ, Phillimore HE. Clinical use of pharmacogenomic tests in 2009. Clin Biochem Rev 2009;30(2):55–65.
20. Herman JS, Easterbrook PJ. The metabolic toxicities of antiretroviral therapy. Int J STD AIDS 2001;12(9):555–62 [quiz 563].
21. Miller KD, Cameron M, Wood LV, et al. Lactic acidosis and hepatic steatosis associated with use of stavudine: report of four cases. Ann Intern Med 2000;133(3):192–6.
22. Brinkman K, Smeitink JA, Romijn JA, et al. Mitochondrial toxicity induced by nucleoside-analogue reverse-transcriptase inhibitors is a key factor in the pathogenesis of antiretroviral-therapy-related lipodystrophy. Lancet 1999;354(9184):1112–5.
23. Calza L, Manfredi R, Chiodo F. Hyperlactataemia and lactic acidosis in HIV-infected patients receiving antiretroviral therapy. Clin Nutr 2005;24(1):5–15.
24. Tan D, Walmsley S, Shen S, et al. Mild to moderate symptoms do not correlate with lactate levels in HIV-positive patients on nucleoside reverse transcriptase inhibitors. HIV Clin Trials 2006;7(3):107–15.
25. Lactic Acidosis International Study Group. Risk factors for lactic acidosis and severe hyperlactataemia in HIV-1-infected adults exposed to antiretroviral therapy. AIDS 2007;21(18):2455–64.
26. Manfredi R, Calza L. HIV infection and the pancreas: risk factors and potential management guidelines. Int J STD AIDS 2008;19(2):99–105.
27. Moore RD, Keruly JC, Chaisson RE. Incidence of pancreatitis in HIV-infected patients receiving nucleoside reverse transcriptase inhibitor drugs. AIDS 2001;15(5):617–20.

28. Moore RD, Fortgang I, Keruly J, et al. Adverse events from drug therapy for human immunodeficiency virus disease. Am J Med 1996;101(1):34–40.

29. Schindzielorz A, Pike I, Daniels M, et al. Rates and risk factors for adverse events associated with didanosine in the expanded access program. Clin Infect Dis 1994;19(6):1076–83.

30. Arenas-Pinto A, Grant AD, Edwards S, et al. Lactic acidosis in HIV infected patients: a systematic review of published cases. Sex Transm Infect 2003; 79(4):340–3.

31. Guaraldi G, Squillace N, Stentarelli C, et al. Nonalcoholic fatty liver disease in HIV-infected patients referred to a metabolic clinic: prevalence, characteristics, and predictors. Clin Infect Dis 2008;47(2):250–7.

32. Carr A, Samaras K, Burton S, et al. A syndrome of peripheral lipodystrophy, hyperlipidaemia and insulin resistance in patients receiving HIV protease inhibitors. AIDS 1998;12(7):F51–8.

33. Dube MP, Johnson DL, Currier JS, et al. Protease inhibitor-associated hyperglycaemia. Lancet 1997;350(9079):713–4.

34. Garg A. Acquired and inherited lipodystrophies. N Engl J Med 2004;350(12): 1220–34.

35. Flexner C. HIV-protease inhibitors. N Engl J Med 1998;338(18):1281–92.

36. Lumpkin M. Reports of diabetes and hyperglycemia in patients receiving protease inhibitors for the treatment of human immunodeficiency virus. In: FDA, editor. Rockville (MD): Public Health Advisory; June 11, 1997.

37. Noor MA, Seneviratne T, Aweeka FT, et al. Indinavir acutely inhibits insulin-stimulated glucose disposal in humans: a randomized, placebo-controlled study. AIDS 2002;16(5):F1–8.

38. Murata H, Hruz PW, Mueckler M. The mechanism of insulin resistance caused by HIV protease inhibitor therapy. J Biol Chem 2000;275(27):20251–4.

39. Zhang S, Carper MJ, Lei X, et al. Protease inhibitors used in the treatment of HIV+ induce beta-cell apoptosis via the mitochondrial pathway and compromise insulin secretion. Am J Physiol Endocrinol Metab 2009;296(4):E925–35.

40. Kaul DR, Cinti SK, Carver PL, et al. HIV protease inhibitors: advances in therapy and adverse reactions, including metabolic complications. Pharmacotherapy 1999;19(3):281–98.

41. Fung HB, Guo Y. Enfuvirtide: a fusion inhibitor for the treatment of HIV infection. Clin Ther 2004;26(3):352–78.

42. Veronese L, Rautaureau J, Sadler BM, et al. Single-dose pharmacokinetics of amprenavir, a human immunodeficiency virus type 1 protease inhibitor, in subjects with normal or impaired hepatic function. Antimicrob Agents Chemother 2000; 44(4):821–6.

43. Friis-Moller N, Sabin CA, Weber R, et al. Combination antiretroviral therapy and the risk of myocardial infarction. N Engl J Med 2003;349(21):1993–2003.

44. Brown TT. Approach to the human immunodeficiency virus-infected patient with lipodystrophy. J Clin Endocrinol Metab 2008;93(8):2937–45.

45. D'Silva M, Leibowitz D, Flaherty JP. Seizure associated with zidovudine. Lancet 1995;346(8972):452.

Postexposure Prophylaxis for HIV

Rachel L. Chin, MD[a,b],*

KEYWORDS

- HIV - PEP - Occupational exposure
- Nonoccupational exposure

Health care workers (HCWs) are at risk for HIV and other infectious pathogens through exposure to blood and body fluids. Antiretroviral medications have been prescribed for postexposure prophylaxis (PEP) following occupational exposure to the human immunodeficiency virus (HIV) since the early 1990s. This practice has since been extended to nonoccupational situations, such as sexual assaults. The efficacy of prophylactic therapy may be highly time-dependent and should be initiated as soon as possible. Wound care management and referral for social, medical, or advocacy services remain important for all cases.

In the United States, it is estimated that between 380,000 and 800,000 hospital-based HCWs sustain sharps injuries annually. It is further estimated that approximately 58% to 73% of needlestick injuries are actually unreported and these national figures do not include nonhospital HCWs, suggesting that current data on sharps injuries significantly underestimate the true number of injuries.[1–3]

RISK OF HIV TRANSMISSION

One of the major concerns about exposures to blood or body fluids is the risk of acquiring an HIV infection. HIV is transmitted primarily through contact with blood, seminal or vaginal fluids, and breast milk. Although HIV can also be recovered from cerebrospinal, synovial, amniotic, peritoneal, pericardial, or pleural fluids, these body fluids are unlikely sources of HIV transmission. Feces, nasal secretions, saliva, sputum, sweat, tears, urine, and vomitus are not considered to be infectious unless they are visibly bloody.[4]

Blood products in the United States have been screened for HIV since the mid-1980s, and the risk of HIV transmission from transfusions is extremely low. The

Disclosures: The author has no disclosures to report.
[a] University of California San Francisco, School of Medicine, San Francisco, CA, USA
[b] Department of Emergency Medicine, San Francisco General Hospital, 1001 Potrero Avenue 1E-21, San Francisco, CA 94110, USA
* Department of Emergency Medicine, San Francisco General Hospital, 1001 Potrero Avenue 1E-21, San Francisco, CA 94110.
E-mail address: Rachel.chin@emergency.ucsf.edu

Emerg Med Clin N Am 28 (2010) 421–429
doi:10.1016/j.emc.2010.01.013
0733-8627/10/$ – see front matter © 2010 Published by Elsevier Inc.

estimated risk of transfusion is 1 infection per 2.6 million transfusion donations.[5] **Table 1** lists the estimated per-act risk for acquisition of HIV by exposure route.

Occupational Exposure

The overall rate of HIV transmission through percutaneous inoculation is reported to be 0.3% (95% confidence interval [CI] 0.2–0.5); the risk of acquiring an HIV infection is greater for percutaneous injuries that involve hollow-bore needles that have been in contact with an artery or vein, when blood is visible on the device, a deep needle-stick, and when the source patient has advanced HIV disease.[6]

Suture needles have not been implicated as a source of infection in prospective studies, but occupational HIV infection has been reported among surgical personnel, and suture needles are 1 potential source of infection.[4,7]

Splashes or infectious material to mucous membranes or broken skin may also transmit HIV infection (estimated risk per exposure, 0.09%; 95% CI 0.006–0.5).[8] Exposure of intact skin to contaminated blood has not been identified as a risk for HIV transmission.[4,7,8]

Nonoccupational Exposure

The risk of HIV transmission from sexual exposure varies according to the nature of the exposure. The estimated risks are 1% to 30% with receptive anal intercourse, 0.1% to 10.0% with insertive anal intercourse and receptive vaginal intercourse, and 0.1% to 1.0% with insertive vaginal intercourse.[9–11] Oral intercourse is considered to pose a lower risk of HIV transmission, although there are case reports of HIV infections in persons where the only reported risk factor was oral intercourse.[12,13] The risks of sexual HIV transmission are difficult to quantify. The risks derive from observational studies and are influenced by many factors, including the presence of genital ulcers, cervical or anal dysplasia, circumcision, the viral load in the genital compartment, and the degree of viral virulence.[10,11] The estimated risk of transmission associated with sharing needles for injection-drug use is approximately 0.67% per needle-sharing contact.[14,15]

Occasionally, a victim presents to the emergency department (ED) after a bite wound and asks about HIV PEP. The risk associated with bite injuries has not been quantified. The victim is usually at low risk unless the biter's saliva is contaminated

Table 1
Estimated per-act risk for acquisition of HIV, by exposure route[a]

Exposure Route	Risk Per 10,000 Exposures to an Infected Source
Blood transfusion	9,000
Needle-sharing injection-drug use	67
Receptive anal intercourse	50
Percutaneous needle stick	30
Receptive penile-vaginal intercourse	10
Insertive anal intercourse	6.5
Insertive penile-vaginal intercourse	10
Receptive oral intercourse	1
Insertive oral intercourse	0.5

[a] Estimates of risk for transmission from sexual exposures assume no condom use.
   Data from CDC. MMRW January 21, 2005;54(RR02):1–20.

with blood. The risk is greater to the biter if blood is drawn from the victim's wound because of exposure to mucous membranes, but the biter is often not the patient who presents to the ED. The estimated risk per exposure can be inferred from the studies examining the risk of occupational exposure from splashes or infectious material to mucous membranes at 0.09%.[8]

The average risk associated with exposure of nonintact skin to HIV-infected fluids and tissues other than blood or bloody fluids is too low to be estimated in prospective studies.[7] Human bite wounds should be treated with standard wound care principles.

TESTING

The types of exposure and medical history of the source patient should guide the decision to start PEP. The use of PEP assumes that the person who was exposed to HIV is not infected with HIV; thus, a negative result of a baseline enzyme-linked immunosorbent assay (ELISA) for antibodies to HIV should be documented concomitantly with the assessment for PEP.[15]

An HIV antibody test can diagnose infections that occurred several weeks or months before, but cannot assess whether the person has been infected recently. Unfortunately, a person recently infected is often highly infectious before the detection of serum antibodies. In occupational settings, a negative highly sensitive rapid ELISA test can rule out the need for PEP. If a rapid test is positive, confirmatory tests should be performed because false positive results can occur. Unless the source patient has risk factors for HIV infection or clinical findings consistent with acute HIV infection such as fever, rash, pharyngitis, lymphadenopathy, and malaise; a quantitative nucleic acid amplification test would be an appropriate test to order. If testing of the source patient in an occupational exposure is delayed for any reason, it is prudent to administer a first dose of PEP pending testing in the source patient.[15]

The source patient in nonoccupational settings is rarely available for testing. Consensus guidelines recommend considering prophylaxis in persons who were exposed to known HIV-infected source patients and to selected high-risk populations, such as men who have sex with men, men who have sex with men and women, commercial sex workers, injection-drug users, history of incarceration, persons from a country where the seroprevalence of HIV is 1% or greater, and persons who have a sexual partner belonging to 1 of these groups. Perpetrators of sexual assault are also considered to be at high risk for being infected with HIV.[15,16]

Hepatitis B and C testing involves examining the source patient's blood for markers of viral infection and for evidence of immunity. Hepatitis B testing assesses for the presence of surface antibody (which indicates immunity to hepatitis B), surface (s) antigen, and envelope (e) antigen (which indicates active viral replication). An ELISA for antibodies against hepatitis C virus (HCV) should be carried out. A follow-up ELISA for antibodies against HIV should be performed at 4 to 6 weeks, 3 months, and 6 months after exposure. Tests for other sexually transmitted diseases should be pursued for nonoccupational exposures if necessary. See **Table 2** for laboratory tests generally recommended for persons after exposure to HIV.

BENEFITS, TIMING AND DURATION OF PEP

PEP should be initiated as soon as possible after exposure to HIV. In the Centers for Disease Control's (CDC) retrospective case-control study of health care personnel, PEP treatment with zidovudine was associated with an 81% reduction (95% CI 43–94) in the risk of HIV infection.[7] Data from clinical trials of prophylaxis against perinatal transmission of HIV consistently demonstrated that antiretroviral therapy (ART) can

Table 2
Regimens for 25-day postexposure prophylaxis for HIV infection.[a]

Regimen	Dose	Daily Pill Burden (no.)[b]	Advantages	Disadvantages
Two-drug Regimens				
Tenofovir-emtricitabine (Truvada)[c]	One tablet (300 mg of tenofovir with 200 mg of emtricitabine) once daily	1	Well tolerated; once-daily dosing	Potential nephrotoxicity
Zidovudine-lamivudine (Combivir)[d]	One tablet (300 mg of zidovudine with 150 mg of lamivudine) once daily	2	Preferred in pregnancy	Twice-daily doling; less well tolerated than tenofovir-emtricitabine (nausea, asthenia, neutropenia, anemia, abnormal liver enzyme levels)
Three-drug Regimens[e]				
Ritonavir-lopinavir (Kaletra) (plus either tenofovir-emtricitabine or zidovudine-lamivudine)	Two tablets (50 mg of ritonavir with 200 mg of lopinavir per tablet) twice daily, or 4 tablets once daily	5 or 6	Either once-daily or twice-daily dosing; 1 copayment; no refrigeration required; most experience in pregnancy; high genetic barrier to resistance	Gastrointestinal side effects such as diarrhea; may cause increased liver enzyme levels or hepatitis

| Ritonavir plus atazanavir (plus either tenofovir-emtricitabine or zidovudine-lamivudine) | 100 mg of ritonavir plus 300 mg of atazanavir once daily | 3 or 4 | Once-daily dosing; well tolerated | Ritonavir must be refrigerated; potential for asymptomatic jaundice, renal stones; may cause increased liver enzyme levels or hepatitis |
| Ritonavir plus darunavir (plus either tenofovir-emtricitabine or zidovudine-lamivudine) | 100 mg of ritonavir plus 2 tablets, each containing 100 mg of darunavir, once daily | 4 or 5 | Once-daily dosing; high genetic barrier to resistance | Ritonavir must be refrigerated; gastrointestinal side effects: may cause increased liver enzyme levels or hepatitis |

a Tenofovir, emtricitabine, and lamivudine all have activity against hepatitis B. Patients with chronic active hepatitis B (ie, patients who are positive for hepatitis B surface antigen) may have flares of hepatitis on withdrawal of these agents at the completion of postexposure prophylaxis treatment. Referral to a hepatitis specialist or serial monthly monitoring of liver enzyme levels for up to 6 months after treatment should be considered.

b The daily pill burden in the 3-drug regimens depends on which 2-drug regimen is chosen.

c The dose of tenofovir-emtricitabine should be reduced to 1 tablet every 48 hours in patients with a creatinine clearance of 30 to 49 mL per minute. Tenofovir-emtricitabine is not recommended in patients with a creatinine clearance of less than 30 mL per minute or in patients who are undergoing hemodialysis; see the guidelines from the Department of Health and Human Services[28] for considerations regarding doses of individual agents in patients with advanced renal dysfunction.

d Zidovudine-lamivudine is not recommended in patients with a creatinine clearance of less than 50 mL per minute; see the guidelines from the Department of Health and Human Services[29] for considerations regarding doses of individual agents in patients with renal dysfunction.

e The boosting agent ritonavir is not considered to be an active drug in tabulating the number of agents in the 3-drug regimen.

Reprinted from Landovitz RJ, Currier JS. Postexposure prophylaxis for HIV infection. N Engl J Med 2009;361:1768-75; with permission. Copyright 2009 Massachusetts Medical Society. All rights reserved.

prevent HIV infection after exposure, even among neonates who are not treated until after birth.[17–20] Data from macaques that were exposed to challenge with simian immunodeficiency virus suggest a greater benefit of PEP when it is initiated within 36 hours after exposure compared with 72 hours after exposure.[15,21,22] PEP should be continued for 28 days, based on the macaque models that demonstrated incomplete protection conferred by shorter courses of PEP.[23]

HIV PEP Regimens

The CDC, Department of Health and Human Services, and the World Health Organization guidelines for prophylaxis after occupational exposure and nonoccupational exposure are available on their Web sites.[16,24–26] In general, the regimens for HIV

Table 3
Laboratory tests generally recommended for persons after exposure to HIV[a]

Test	Recommended During Treatment		Recommended at Follow-up		
	Baseline	Symptom-directed[b]	4–6 weeks	12 weeks	24 weeks
ELISA for HIV antibodies	Yes	Yes	Yes	Yes	Yes
Creatinine, liver function, and complete blood count with differential count	Yes	Yes	No	No	No
HIV viral load	No	Yes	No	No	No
Anti-HBs antibodies	Yes[c]	No	No	No	No
HBsAg	Yes[c,d]	No	No	No	No
HCV antibodies	Yes	No	Yes	Yes	Yes
HCV RNA1[e]	No	Yes	Yes	Yes	Yes
Screening, including rapid plasma reagin test, for other sexually transmitted infections[f]	Yes	Yes	No	Yes	No

[a] Patients who receive zidovudine plus lamivudine-based regimens should have a complete blood count and measurement of liver enzyme levels at 2 weeks of treatment, irrespective of the presence or absence of clinical symptoms. Tenofovir plus emtricitabine-based regimens generally involve few side effects, and symptom-directed assessment of serum creatinine or liver enzyme levels should be considered. The addition of a ritonavir-boosted protease inhibitor should be followed by symptom-directed assessment of liver enzyme levels, serum glucose levels, or both. Anti-HBs antibodies denotes hepatitis B virus surface antibodies; ELISA, enzyme-linked immunosorbent assay; HBsAg, hepatitis B surface antigen; HCV, hepatitis C virus.
[b] Symptom-directed tests are for signs or symptoms of toxic effects (rash, nausea, vomiting, or abdominal pain) or HIV seroconversion (fever, fatigue, lymphadenopathy, rash, or oral or genital ulcers).
[c] If tests for anti-HBs antibodies and HBsAg are both negative, a vaccination series against HBV infection should be initiated and completed.
[d] If the patient is HBsAg positive, they should have monthly follow-up of liver function tests after discontinuation of postexposure prophylactic regimens containing tenofovir, lamivudine, or emtricitabine; referral to a specialist in viral hepatitis should tie considered.
[e] HCV RNA testing may identify early HCV seroconversion; early detection and treatment during acute HCV infection may avert or ameliorate chronic disease. *Data from* Dienstag and McHutchison.[30]
[f] Rapid plasma reagin testing and testing of urethral-swab and rectal-swab specimens for gonorrhea and chlamydia and of pharyngeal-swab specimens for gonorrhea should be performed as appropriate, according to the patient's sexual risk-taking behaviors and the type of exposure to HIV.

Table 4	
Resources for managing exposure to blood and body fluids	
Resource	**Contact Information**
National Clinicians' Postexposure Prophylaxis hotline (PEPline)	+1 888 448 4911
Needlestick! (online decision-making support for clinicians)	http://www.needlestick.mednet.ucla.edu
CDC hepatitis information line	+1 888 443 7232 http://www.cdc.gov/hepatitis
Perinatal HIV hotline	+1 888 448 8765
AIDS treatment info	http://www.hivatis.org

PEP consist of 2 nucleotide or nucleoside reverse transcriptase inhibitors for the basic regimen and the addition of a protease inhibitor or nonnucleoside reverse transcriptase inhibitor for the expanded regimen. Nevirapine should not be used for PEP because it has been associated with fatal hepatic and dermatologic toxicities in patients not infected with HIV.[27] Treatment is recommended for 28 days, unless the source is found to be uninfected, or severe adverse side effects occur. See **Table 3** for regimens for PEP for HIV infection.

SUMMARY

EDs should have protocols that facilitate rapid testing and consultations. Emergency physicians can seek expert consultation advice on occupational or nonoccupational exposures to HIV from the 24-hour National Clinicians' Postexposure Prophylaxis Hotline (PEPline) at (+1 888 448 4911). See **Table 4** for resources for managing exposure to blood and body fluids.

REFERENCES

1. Alvarado-Ramy F, Beltrami EM, Short LJ, et al. A comprehensive approach to percutaneous injury prevention during phlebotomy: results of a multicenter study, 1993-1995. Infect Control Hosp Epidemiol 2003;24(2):97–104.
2. Dement JM, Epling C, Ostbye T, et al. Blood and body fluid exposure risks among health care workers: results from the Duke Health and Safety Surveillance System. Am J Ind Med 2004;46(6):637–48.
3. Perry JPG, Jagger J. EPINet report: 2007 percutaneous injury rates. 2009. International Healthcare Worker Safety. Available at: www.healthsystem.virginia.edu/internet/epinet/EPINet-2007-rates.pdf. Accessed November 9, 2009.
4. US Public Health Service. Updated US Public Health Service guidelines for the management of occupational exposures to HBV, HCV, and HIV and recommendations for postexposure prophylaxis. MMWR Recomm Rep 2001;50(RR-11):1–52.
5. Lackritz EM, Satten GA, Aberle-Grasse J, et al. Estimated risk of transmission of the human immunodeficiency virus by screened blood in the United States. N Engl J Med 1995;333(26):1721–5.
6. Cardo DM, Culver DH, Ciesielski CA, et al. A case-control study of HIV seroconversion in health care workers after percutaneous exposure. Centers for Disease Control and Prevention Needlestick Surveillance Group. N Engl J Med 1997;337(21):1485–90.

7. Gerberding JL. Clinical practice. Occupational exposure to HIV in health care settings. N Engl J Med 2003;348(9):826–33.

8. Ippolito G, Puro V, De Carli G. The risk of occupational human immunodeficiency virus infection in health care workers. Italian Multicenter Study. The Italian Study Group on Occupational Risk of HIV infection. Arch Intern Med 1993;153(12): 1451–8.

9. Centers for Disease Control and Prevention. Antiretroviral postexposure prophylaxis after sexual, injection drug use, or other nonoccupational exposure to HIV in the United States: recommendations from the U.S. Department of Health and Human Services. Atlanta (GA): Centers for Disease Control and Prevention; 2005.

10. Powers KA, Poole C, Pettifor AE, et al. Rethinking the heterosexual infectivity of HIV-1: a systematic review and meta-analysis. Lancet Infect Dis 2008;8(9): 553–63.

11. Boily MC, Baggaley RF, Wang L, et al. Heterosexual risk of HIV-1 infection per sexual act: systematic review and meta-analysis of observational studies. Lancet Infect Dis 2009;9(2):118–29.

12. Lifson AR, O'Malley PM, Hessol NA, et al. HIV seroconversion in two homosexual men after receptive oral intercourse with ejaculation: implications for counseling concerning safe sexual practices. Am J Public Health 1990;80(12):1509–11.

13. Rozenbaum W, Gharakhanian S, Cardon B, et al. HIV transmission by oral sex. Lancet 1988;1(8599):1395.

14. Kaplan EH, Heimer R. HIV incidence among New Haven needle exchange participants: updated estimates from syringe tracking and testing data. J Acquir Immune Syndr Hum Retrovirol 1995;10:175–6.

15. Landovitz RJ, Currier JS. Clinical practice. Postexposure prophylaxis for HIV infection. N Engl J Med 2009;361(18):1768–75.

16. Smith DK, Grohskopf LA, Black RJ, et al. Antiretroviral postexposure prophylaxis after sexual, injection-drug use, or other nonoccupational exposure to HIV in the United States: recommendations from the U.S. Department of Health and Human Services. MMWR Recomm Rep 2005;54(RR-2):1–20.

17. Kuhn L, Stein ZA. Mother-to-infant HIV transmission: timing, risk factors and prevention. Paediatr Perinat Epidemiol 1995;9(1):1–29.

18. Connor EM, Sperling RS, Gelber R, et al. Reduction of maternal-infant transmission of human immunodeficiency virus type 1 with zidovudine treatment. Pediatric AIDS Clinical Trials Group Protocol 076 Study Group. N Engl J Med 1994;331(18): 1173–80.

19. Sperling RS, Shapiro DE, Coombs RW, et al. Maternal viral load, zidovudine treatment, and the risk of transmission of human immunodeficiency virus type 1 from mother to infant. Pediatric AIDS Clinical Trials Group Protocol 076 Study Group. N Engl J Med 1996;335(22):1621–9.

20. Guay LA, Musoke P, Fleming T, et al. Intrapartum and neonatal single-dose nevirapine compared with zidovudine for prevention of mother-to-child transmission of HIV-1 in Kampala, Uganda: HIVNET 012 randomised trial. Lancet 1999; 354(9181):795–802.

21. Tsai CC, Follis KE, Sabo A, et al. Prevention of SIV infection in macaques by (R)-9-(2-phosphonylmethoxypropyl)adenine. Science 1995;270(5239):1197–9.

22. Otten RA, Smith DK, Adams DR, et al. Efficacy of postexposure prophylaxis after intravaginal exposure of pig-tailed macaques to a human-derived retrovirus (human immunodeficiency virus type 2). J Virol 2000;74(20):9771–5.

23. Tsai CC, Emau P, Follis KE, et al. Effectiveness of postinoculation (R)-9-(2-phosphonylmethoxypropyl) adenine treatment for prevention of persistent simian

immunodeficiency virus SIVmne infection depends critically on timing of initiation and duration of treatment. J Virol 1998;72(5):4265–73.

24. Panlilio AL, Cardo DM, Grohskopf LA, et al. Updated U.S. Public Health Service guidelines for the management of occupational exposures to HIV and recommendations for postexposure prophylaxis. MMWR Recomm Rep 2005;54(RR-9):1–17.

25. Notice to Readers Updated information regarding antiretroviral agents used as HIV postexposure prophylaxis for occupational HIV exposures. MMWR Morb Mortal Wkly Rep 2007;56(49):1291–2.

26. World Health Organization. Post-exposure prophylaxis to prevent HIV infection: joint WHO/ILO guidelines on post-exposure prophylaxis (PEP) to prevent HIV infection. Geneva (Switzerland): World Health Organization; 2007.

27. From the Centers for Disease Control and Prevention. Serious adverse events attributed to nevirapine regimens for postexposure prophylaxis after HIV exposures–worldwide, 1997-2000. JAMA 2001;285(4):402–3.

28. Guidelines for the use of antiretroviral agents in HIV-1-infected adults and adolescents. Washington, DC: Department of Health and Human Services; 2008. Available at: http://www.aidsinfo.nih.gov/contentfiles/AdultandAdolescentGL.pdf. Accessed November 9, 2009.

29. Mayer KH, Mimiaga MJ, Cohen D, et al. Tenofovir DF plus lamivudine or emtricitabine for nonoccupational postexposure prophylaxis (NPEP) in a Boston Community Health Center. J Acquir Immune Defic Syndr 2008;47(4):494–9.

30. Dienstag JL, McHutchison JG. American Gastroenterological Association technical review on the management of hepatitis C. Gastroenterology 2006;130(1): 231–64 [quiz: 214–37].

Index

Note: Page numbers of article titles are in **boldface** type.

A

Emerg Med Clin N Am 28 (2010) 431–438
doi:10.1016/S0733-8627(10)00026-X
0733-8627/10/$ – see front matter © 2010 Elsevier Inc. All rights reserved.

emed.theclinics.com

Moving?

Make sure your subscription moves with you!

To notify us of your new address, find your **Clinics Account Number** (located on your mailing label above your name), and contact customer service at:

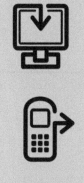

Email: journalscustomerservice-usa@elsevier.com

800-654-2452 (subscribers in the U.S. & Canada)
314-447-8871 (subscribers outside of the U.S. & Canada)

Fax number: 314-447-8029

**Elsevier Health Sciences Division
Subscription Customer Service
3251 Riverport Lane
Maryland Heights, MO 63043**

*To ensure uninterrupted delivery of your subscription, please notify us at least 4 weeks in advance of move.

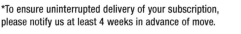

Printed and bound by CPI Group (UK) Ltd, Croydon, CR0 4YY

03/10/2024

01040453-0016